Louise Roddon is a respected journalist specialising in health and lifestyle topics. Her articles have appeared in *The Times*, the *Daily Mail*, *Today*, the *Evening Standard* and the *European* as well as many leading magazines. She is the author of *Am I a Monster or is this PMS?*, another title in the Headline Health Kicks series.

She has changed from being a keen fan of good wine, rich foods, cigarettes and a lazy lifestyle to someone who now exercises regularly, eats properly, sleeps well and still has a great sense of humour!

Jacky Fleming is a best-selling cartoonist. Her books, *Be a Bloody Train Driver*, *Never Give Up*, *Falling in Love* and *Dear Katie* are published by Penguin.

GW00801661

Also by Louise Roddon

Am I a Monster or is this PMS?: Self help for PMS sufferers

SKIN DEEP

Self help for healthy skin

Louise Roddon

HEADLINE

First published in 1995
by HEADLINE BOOK PUBLISHING

10 9 8 7 6 5 4 3 2 1

ISBN 0 7472 5122 3

Typeset by
Letterpart Limited, Reigate, Surrey

Printed and bound in Great Britain by
Cox & Wyman Ltd, Reading, Berks

HEADLINE BOOK PUBLISHING
A division of Hodder Headline PLC
338 Euston Road
London NW1 3BH

This book is dedicated to David – with my love

Acknowledgements

I would like to thank Ashley Medicks for all his help and advice. I am also indebted to all those people who provided their experiences as case studies for this book.

Contents

Preface

WHAT IS SKIN?

Skin: most people never give it a second thought – unless, of course, something goes wrong with it. For many, the skin is little more than a human-sized 'envelope' – something to keep our outsides out, and our insides safely sealed in. But our skin is incredibly important. It is our largest organ, covering between fifteen and twenty square feet; it weighs around ten pounds, and it is like some marvellous washable, waterproof coat which can also function as a temperature regulator, a self-healer and a waste eliminator: if only clothes were so efficient!

Skin is designed to be tough, yet it also has to be sensitive to what's going on around us. And, when things go wrong on the inside, the skin acts like a mirror, its colour and texture reflecting back the state of our health.

'Pale as a ghost', 'sweating like a pig', 'thick-skinned', 'in the pink' – when you think about it, we often describe how people seem to us, by the condition and colour of their skin. In fact, there are very few conditions, both physical and indeed psychological, which do not reflect themselves in the state of our skin.

We live in polluted stressful times, and so it shouldn't

really surprise us that millions of people suffer from skin disorders. And they are on the increase – from the humble outbreak of temporary pimples to the more persistent chronic conditions like eczema and psoriasis. If you are a skin sufferer, you will also probably be aware already that skin disorders have a vastly lower profile than say heart disease in this country; perhaps you have waited for months to see a dermatologist, only to be allowed a few minutes' consultation, once your appointment comes through. Dermatology is hugely underfunded in the UK, and in desperation, most sufferers tend to resort to treating their symptoms with prescribed orthodox drugs like steroids and antibiotics. Short term, these can of course be very helpful – but far better is to take time to address the cause of the problem, to work out why the skin is not functioning healthily in the first place: good health is more than skin deep!

This book is for anyone whose life has been affected by a skin problem. Whether it be a dry, flaky skin condition that hits you only in winter months, or chronic recurring acne – even the odd twinge of concern about the onslaught of wrinkles has its place in *Skin Deep*. Stress, a poor self-image, emotional problems – not to mention the fear of 'going public', of facing other people's possible rejection when your skin problem is visible: all these take their toll on your general well-being, and the well-being of your skin. In Part Two, we look at ways you can help yourself, and tackle the root cause of your problem.

HOW DOES SKIN WORK?

The skin is made up of three distinct layers: the epidermis, the dermis, and the subcutaneous fat layer.

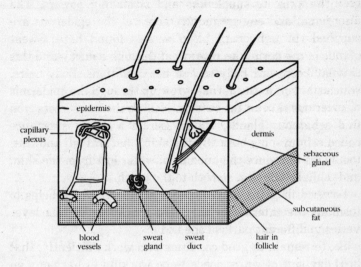

The epidermis is the top, outer layer of the skin. It's the part of the skin you can see, and is thickest on those parts that experience the most friction – for example, the soles of your feet and the palms of your hands. At its base, new skin cells are continually being made, and this causes older cells to be pushed to the surface. The dry dead cells on the surface of the skin stick loosely together and form a waterproof scaly layer, which helps protect the new cells beneath them. That scaly layer also keeps water in our skin, and germs and infections on the outside.

The dermis is the thick elastic middle section of skin. It is the solid ground on which the 'wall' of the epidermis is built. It contains nerves which give us our touch and pain sensations, and collagen and elastin which hold the dermis and the epidermis to the rest of the body by tiny threads, and give the skin its suppleness and stretching powers. The nutritional and energy requirements of the epidermis are supplied through small blood vessels found here. Sweat glands in the dermis secrete sweat through a duct – and this is what keeps our body cool in hot conditions. Body hairs, which start off in the dermis, grow up through the epidermis to cover our skin on the outside. Next to the hairs' roots, you find sebaceous glands, which secrete a sticky substance called sebum – it's basically the skin's natural oil, and this, too, helps to reduce the amount of water lost from the skin, and to make the skin smooth to the touch.

Lower still is the subcutaneous fat layer, which helps to insulate the internal organs. The thickness of this layer varies in different parts of the body.

So, to remain in good condition and work efficiently, that birthday suit of yours needs to be working in harmony on every level! When things get out of balance, those problems start.

What to avoid

Certain factors can be pinpointed as enemies to healthy skin. Poor nutrition and too much alcohol (see Chapter 7); the sun (see Chapter 6) and stress (see Chapter 12). Antibiotics can affect some skin conditions adversely, even though they are also prescribed for certain problems, such as **acne**. Smoking, however, never did anyone's skin any good, quite apart from all the wrinkles it can give you . . .

PART 1

Identifying your skin problem

CHAPTER 1

Bacterial Skin Infections

BOILS AND ABSCESSES

We've seen what a staggeringly versatile set-up the skin is – but sometimes even the best, most complex bits of wizardry can break down. Even though we all have bacteria living happily away on our bodies, occasionally the nasties manage to invade, and then it's showtime! And as all you skin sufferers will know, infection has nothing to do with lack of cleanliness, with being dirty. Often, as with eczema sufferers, people with skin infections wash too much for their own good – but more of that later in the book.

What is a boil?
At the risk of sounding like something out of an ancient war film or a B horror movie, this is what happens when bacterial infection attacks.

The epidermis is like the body's 'front line'. This outer layer of skin defends the body against disease-forming bacteria. When this barrier breaks down, nasty and incredibly single-minded bacteria spring into action, ready to invade and wreak havoc. Any cracked, scratched and cut bit of skin is at risk – but the body is no fool, even in its weakened state. Once those germs have made their entry, the body's army of fighters, its immune system, gets to work, pumping blood into the problem area. The skin tissue starts to change its usual regime, and alters its cell structure, thus 'highlighting' the trouble spot, if you will excuse the pun – and the result is a boil.

It is that boost in blood supply which causes the skin to swell, go red and increase in heat. When that skin gets stretched, you get pain, and if the inflammation is slow to heal, pus (a mixture of bacteria, white cells and blood fluids) can form in the centre of the boil.

What causes a boil?

But why is the boil there in the first place? As with other skin infections (**abscesses, impetigo, cold sores**) the appearance of a boil may be a sign that you are run down and tired. Sometimes they occur because of poor diet. Boils are basically deeper seated infections of the hair follicle than in ordinary spots or acne and start out as tender red lumps. Their appear-ance is a way of letting you know that your immune system isn't its usual fighting fit self. If you're getting them regularly, you should have a proper check up with your doctor as recurrence can be an indicator of diabetes mellitus.

Boils, though uncomfortable, are really only minor infections of the skin. You probably think they are disfiguring and utterly enormous, but very rarely is that the case. We live in a face and figure focused society, so changes in the appearance of your skin can be very upsetting – especially, as with boils, when the skin condition is accompanied by pain. But rest assured, there are plenty of cures available, and if you can be courageous enough to let time take the lead and leave the boil alone, that pus will eventually come to a head, breaking through the surface of the skin and dispersing – taking with it all that throbbing pain and infection. Squeeze the boil, and you risk infecting the area with bacteria, which could leave a scar – it will also be very painful indeed. However, a small boil is more comfortable if protected; when it is just about to 'point', it can be pierced with a clean needle, and the pus gently let out. But be very careful with boils on the face – these should always get medical attention.

What is an abscess?

Abscesses are closely related to boils, in that essentially they are boils gone wrong! When the pus in the head of the boil remains in the skin, and gets trapped in a cavity, it is called an abscess. And if the boil becomes large, with several pus-filled heads, this is called a carbuncle. Abscesses or carbuncles really require medical supervision – they may need to be treated with antibiotics, and lanced and drained. Again, your doctor will advise you.

Boils and abscesses: how you can help yourself

• Look at your intake of vitamins and minerals. Consider boosting your immune system (Chapter 8) with vitamin C and beta carotene.
• Don't touch the boil or abscess too much, and certainly don't try to squeeze it.
• Consider long-term action: stress relief, a better diet, giving up bad habits like smoking or drinking too much.
• Some herbal remedies may help. We discuss these in Chapter 10.

IMPETIGO

Although impetigo is more common with children, I got impetigo two years ago at the ripe old age of thirty-seven!

My face erupted into tiny boil-like red spots which were sore and itchy. They then developed blistery heads which crusted over – all tremendously attractive and confidence boosting, as you can imagine! People talked to my spots and not to my face, and my instinct was to drench them in camouflaging concealer, until my doctor advised me against this. The spots were persistent little so-and-sos. I was prescribed a local antibiotic ointment, but I found this impossibly sticky stuff, which eventually only increased the itchiness. A change-over to an antibiotic cream eventually did the trick – but I know that I had been run down and depressed before they appeared, and lazy too, about eating properly and healthily – so you may want to look at your life-style if you think impetigo is your problem.

What is impetigo?
● Impetigo is a bacterial skin infection.
● It is common in warm weather when the skin is more prone to sweating, and bacteria are easily spread from one patch to another.
● It occurs on the face, lips and around the nose.
● It is highly contagious and spreads rapidly.
● Sufferers have sore red spots with blistery weepy heads which ooze sticky fluid, leaving yellow crusty scabs.

What causes impetigo?
It is caused by the streptococcus and staphylococcus bacteria entering the skin through a cut. Some people naturally harbour the disease-producing strain of these bacteria in their nostrils – and from there, it can spread to infect a cut or scratch.

Impetigo: how you can help yourself
- Be really vigilant about using clean pillowslips, face cloths and towels, and boil after use. Don't share with others, since impetigo is highly contagious.
- Wash loose crusts off with unperfumed soap and warm water.
- Try and avoid wearing make-up. Curing is through topical application of creams (that means applying the cream directly onto the infected area), so cosmetics will only mess up the healing process, and you could spread the infection to your make-up and thus reinfect yourself.
- Look at your diet. (See Chapter 7.) Also, you may be low in supplements like vitamin C, beta carotene or zinc. (Chapter 8 will help here.)
- Consider homeopathic cures if you don't fancy using antibiotics; they work for some people. We discuss relevant ones in Chapter 11.
- Above all, consider your life-style and stress levels. Learn to relax! Chapter 12 points the way to a healthier, happier you.

CHAPTER 2

Viral Skin Conditions

COLD SORES

Sarah's story

'OK, so I've not got the best skin in the world, but I look after it as well as I can. Where it causes me problems is when a cold sore appears – usually at the most inappropriate times. I don't know if this is an established stress-related condition, but my last attack would indicate so. I hadn't had a boyfriend for years, and finally friends introduced me to someone I really liked – not the usual match-making disaster where they get it completely wrong! Anyway, I liked Andy, and he seemed to like me. He knew where I worked, so there was none of that embarrassing "How can I give him my phone number, without appearing pushy" nonsense. The trouble was, I didn't hear from him for three weeks, and my confidence plummeted. I chastised myself for assuming he liked me. I got mopey, smoked too much, got flu and ended up with a ruddy great scabby cold sore right on top of my upper lip. Wouldn't you know it, that's when he chose to ring! His mother had been ill and he'd had to go back to Scotland. I put him off for a few days, but I was really keen to see him. The sore was at its medieval black plague stage by the time of our first date. I tried to laugh it off, but he didn't kiss me goodnight! Oh! for all you cold sore sufferers out there – the sore disappeared and Andy and I are very much an item. Apparently I didn't scare him off!'

What are cold sores?

Cold sores are the real 'ouch' of viral skin infections, but apart from the soreness, this is not a serious condition. The problems it causes have more to do with the embarrassment and self-consciousness which plague the sufferer, since most cold sores hit the mouth area first and foremost, as Sarah explained so vividly!

The four stages of an attack

1. **The Tingle Factor**: when your skin starts to itch and tingle, it's usually a sign that there's a cold sore on its way. Often this is the best moment to apply an anti-viral ointment or cream (for example, Zovirax) to help shorten the life of the cold sore.
2. **Blisters**: a small raised 'spot' swells to form blisters. These are very often painful.
3. **The Weepies**: this is the embarrassing, uncomfortable and contagious point in the life of a cold sore. The blisters collapse and join together to form one large weeping sore.
4. **Scab Stage**: as the blisters dry out, so they begin to heal. A scab starts to grow. Don't touch or pick! It will crack and bleed and be very painful indeed.

Healing

The cold sore can take ten or more days to heal if left to its own devices. But there are ways you can speed up the process. (See page 12.)

What causes cold sores?
Cold sores are caused by the herpes simplex type I or type II
viruses. These are from the herpes group of viruses, others of
which cause glandular fever, shingles, as we shall see, and
chickenpox.

Who gets cold sores?
A staggering 12 million people in the UK get cold sores on a
regular basis – that's one in five poor sufferers under attack
from two to ten times a year. The important (and rather
depressing) thing about cold sores is that after your first
infection, you may always be prone to them, even though the
virus can lie dormant for years. You usually get infected in
early childhood – for instance, after being kissed by someone
with the infection. The virus passes into the skin, and travels
up a nerve, where it hides in the nerve junction waiting to be
activated. This first attack can often be symptomless,
though from here on in, certain conditions can trigger off an
infection. These are:

- being run down
- exposure to sunlight
- colds and flu
- menstruation
- a physical injury
- tiredness
- a stomach upset
- stress and emotional upset

If this sounds too horribly like a profile of your 'normal'
physical self (tired, moody, premenstrual and with a runny
nose!) rest assured that with each new attack, the body is
making more antibodies to fight the cold sore. That means

11

that in time, outbreaks should become less severe, and even less frequent.

To kiss or not to kiss
Bear in mind, though, that when you've got a cold sore, that sore will be highly contagious, especially at the 'weeping' stage – not you, that is, but the blisters! You should avoid kissing and close physical contact with others, unless you want to make yourself very unpopular! Keep your kisses till the blisters have gone, which usually means abstaining for a week.

You can also infect other parts of your own body, especially where there is broken skin, if you have been touching the cold sore and haven't washed your hands afterwards. Be particularly vigilant you don't rub your eyes after touching your cold sore. And if you are a mother with a young baby, be particularly careful because the very young are extremely susceptible to the virus.

Cold sores: how you can help yourself
● Apply an anti-viral ointment or cream bought from a chemist as soon as you feel the tingle. Your chemist will advise which one to choose.
● Apply the treatment cream to the affected area every four or so hours, and make sure you wash your hands both before and afterwards. Keep reapplying for five days.
● An old wives' remedy, which seems to work for some, is to dab cold coffee (yes, really!) onto the area with gauze or clean cotton wool and allow to dry. Repeat this every two hours.
● Always keep the cold sore dry and clean.
● Don't pick at the scab, and generally try not to touch the cold sore except to apply ointment.

• If you're prone to cold sores, always keep a treatment cream in the medicine chest. Early treatment is vital.

• Look to your diet, and make sure it is well balanced. Keep your vitamin C levels up. Look, too, to any stresses in your life. If you are the outdoors type, use a good sunblock on the mouth area.

• At the risk of making you feel like some plague ridden so-and-so, it really is advisable during an attack to keep all your eating and drinking utensils, your flannels, and towels away from family members, and make sure they are scrupulously cleaned.

• Avoid bright sunlight and cold wind.

• Change your toothbrush regularly, as this can carry the virus.

SHINGLES

Fiona's story

'Stress does funny things to you, doesn't it? Bob and I were really looking forward to getting married – but as with many other couples, the ceremony got stage-managed by our mothers right from day one, and though we had wanted a fairly quiet do with just immediate family and close friends, suddenly, all these unknown aunts were returning their RSVPs through the post. I felt completely helpless and got very ratty in the weeks leading up to the wedding. Well, that just made me feel worse about everything, because Bob seemed so calm, and there I was, shouting and screaming all over the place! I kept on asking Bob how he was feeling – was he nervous, or regretting marrying me? He just said he felt fine, and was having no problems with the idea of getting married. Well, would you believe it. Two weeks before the

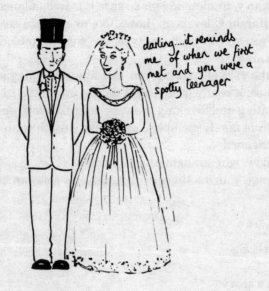

darling....it reminds me of when we first met and you were a spotty teenager

Big Day, he had a nasty outbreak of shingles. If that's not nerves, I don't know what is!'

As Fiona's story shows, shingles is one of those skin conditions that can be exacerbated by stress and worry. Bob wasn't 'expressing' what after all are natural fears about getting married – so effectively, his skin did the job for him.

What are shingles?
Shingles are caused by a different strain of the herpes virus that triggers **cold sores**, known as the Varicella zoster virus. This virus is also responsible for chickenpox, so anyone who gets hit with an attack of shingles, will have had

chickenpox sometime in the past, even if he or she was unaware of it. Sometimes you can get what are called 'sub-clinical attacks' of chickenpox, where no actual spots appear. If the immune system is not at its strongest, due to age or stress, the virus can be activated again to cause not chickenpox this time, but shingles.

Shingles are also different in appearance from chickenpox. The condition is characterised by a rash of blisters on the skin – frequently accompanied by severe stinging pain. In fact, the pain is often the first symptom of an attack of shingles, and can last after the rash has disappeared. A few days later, and the rash appears in the region where the pain is – and this will eventually blister and scab over. The most common area of attack is around your rib region, forming into something looking a bit like a belt. Old wives' tales used to warn that if the rash met in the middle, it would be fatal – rest assured that's a load of baloney! The rash normally clears after a few weeks.

What causes shingles?
A history of chickenpox notwithstanding, Fiona's story reveals that all manner of events can trigger an attack of shingles – but the most common circumstances are:

● if you are exhausted – both physically and emotionally
● if you have had an illness – i.e. if your body's defence mechanisms are 'down'

Who gets shingles?
The older you are, the more likely that you will have developed shingles at some point. A study of people in their eighties revealed that at least one in two had suffered the condition.

15

Shingles: how you can help yourself
• Early treatment is the best course if you want to shorten the attack and make it less severe. Before the rash appears, try an over-the-counter anti-viral cream like Zovirax, which is excellent if taken early enough.
• Calamine lotion can be very soothing at the stinging stage.
• If you are worried, see your GP who may prescribe tablets to lessen and shorten the attack.
• Keep the skin clean. If germs get to infect the blisters, it could lead to scarring.
• Try to avoid stresses in your life. Learn to unwind, and relax.
• Look at your diet. You are probably run down, so make sure that what you are eating is nutritious. Supplements like zinc and vitamin C can be helpful – and our chapter on nutrition will point you towards those foods you should avoid.
• Homeopathic treatment can help. Remedies like Arsenicum can soothe when the skin erupts, and Rhus tox. will help with the itching and pain.
• Herbal remedies, when administered correctly and professionally, have been shown to help. St John's wort, passion flower, skullcap, echinacea and valerian are the herbs recommended for strengthening nerve cells. Use either as a bath or as a tonic. Also, Traditional Chinese Medicine can work wonders – see Chapter 9.

WARTS AND VERRUCAS

Warts – the very name conjures up images of skinny-looking women in pointy hats, a gnarled hand covered in warts as

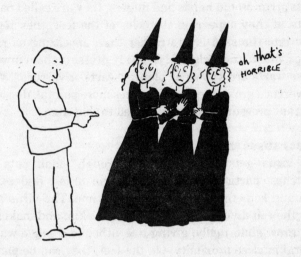

oh that's HORRIBLE

they dole out their words of doom. Ugly-looking toads dispensing warts to the wicked spring to mind, and an equally bizarre collection of old wives' tales for curing them.

In the olden days, people ignorantly associated warts with forces of evil, witches and warlocks – and sure, they're not the most attractive of skin conditions to acquire – but getting them doesn't mean you're a bad person! One old-fashioned 'cure' was to rub your warts with stones. You then wrapped the stones up and left them at the crossroads on the way to church. If someone passing by picked up the stones, he or she would heal your warts by getting infected themselves!

What are warts?
Very simply, warts are small raised dry bumps or nodules of skin which can appear on the hands, face and knees. Again,

the cause is down to a viral attack on the skin cells. When warts occur on the hands and fingers, they are called palmar warts. If they appear on the soles of the feet, they tend to grow into the skin layers rather than appearing as raised lumps, due to the weight of the body pressing them inwards. These warts are known as plantar warts or verrucas. When the verruca grows larger, it becomes more painful, due to the constant pressure of weight applied to that area.

What causes them?

The virus gets into the skin through small cuts and scratches, particularly in moist warm areas, and can lie dormant, sometimes for months at a time. The virus takes over the cell division mechanism of the skin, and makes the skin grow abnormally, giving rise either to a single wart or several in close proximity. On the feet, they can be painful, but ordinary warts that occur on your hands rarely hurt. It can't be stressed enough that warts are harmless – and if you leave them alone, most will disappear of their own accord, albeit over a lengthy period of time.

Who gets them?

Warts and verrucas are transmitted from person to person, and verrucas in particular can frequently attack children, who are used to running around in bare feet. Some people are more prone to warts than others, depending on their immunity to the wart virus, and their resistance to infection.

Genital warts, which are caused by a different strain of the wart virus, are most commonly sexually transmitted. These are usually small and you may have many of them at once. They will require a different kind of treatment, and you should consult your GP.

Warts and verrucas: how you can help yourself
If you find warts unsightly, you need to treat them every day
with a solution or cream which you can buy in any chemist.
Those containing salicylic acid will soften the wart and
loosen it. The wart can then be pared down.

● Wart and verruca treatments contain caustic substances, so make sure they don't come into contact with
healthy skin, since they can make the surrounding skin
feel very sore indeed. Immediately wash off any solution to
avoid painful burns, or cover the surrounding healthy skin
with Vaseline.
● If you have a wart that doesn't respond to over-the-
counter treatments, or if it bleeds or enlarges, seek your
GP's advice. It may be that the wart needs to be frozen off
with liquid nitrogen, though this method is not suitable for
small children, because it is painful and can cause blistering.
● Try essential tea tree oil, which has a strong anti-viral
element.
● Verrucas are treated in much the same way as warts,
though you need only use the treatment two or three times
a week. A felt corn plaster can make the treatment less
painful, by taking the pressure of weight off the verruca.
Enlarge the hole in the plaster by snipping with scissors,
and cover the verruca with a waterproof plaster after
treatment.
● When the verruca looks soft and spongy, remove the
plasters and let the skin 'breathe' – it should now be ready to
drop off.
● When you first get warts, remember that they spread
easily – so use your own towels.
● To swim or not to swim? Verrucas thrive in a warm

moist environment, but some doctors think there is no need for a child with a verruca to avoid swimming. Just make sure the verruca is covered with a waterproof plaster to avoid it spreading to others and to protect it from dirt and the possibility of grazing its surface.

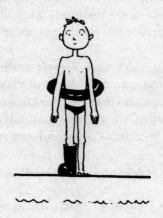

CHAPTER 3

Moist and Fungal Skin Conditions

ATHLETE'S FOOT, RINGWORM AND NAPPY RASH

Warm, moist and sweaty . . . sounds utterly disgusting, doesn't it? But these are precisely the three very natural bodily states that are needed in order for fungal skin conditions to thrive. We all sweat, we all get hot – we all wear shoes and sometimes clothes that are too tight for us – and as a result, we are all prone to outbreaks of athlete's foot and ringworm – even if nappy rash may have now passed us by!

What is athlete's foot?
This is a common fungal skin infection, and unfortunately, once contracted, it can be hard to get rid of. No – you won't suddenly develop the skills of a long-distance runner or TV gladiator, but you will know when you've got athlete's foot if the skin between your toes starts to itch uncontrollably. The skin might crack, become soggy and get very sore. Sometimes it will peel, exposing very pink and tender skin underneath. Occasionally blisters appear.

What causes it?
Athlete's foot is associated with wearing shoes and having

sweaty feet. It can be picked up in gyms, changing rooms and showers.

Athlete's foot: how you can help yourself
• You must treat athlete's foot immediately, since it is easy to pass on to other people.
• There are plenty of anti-fungal products which can be readily obtained from your local chemist. Creams like Canesten and powders like Mycil are very effective, and need to be applied at least twice daily until the skin returns to its normal state.
• Make sure you keep your feet clean and dry at all times. At home, try 'airing' them, by going without restricting shoes or socks. If you are walking in public areas, try wearing sandals.
• Keep the feet cool, wherever possible.
• Wash stockings and socks daily.
• Sprinkle anti-fungal powder liberally onto the feet and in between the toes. You can dust your socks and shoes too, which will help combat sweating.
• If you get infection on your toe nails, pharmaceutical products such as Loceryl may help. This is the trade name of an anti-fungal paint, available on prescription from your GP, which is said to be more safe and effective than the usual course of taking antibiotic tablets. Loceryl will work much more quickly than oral antibiotics.
• Continue any treatment for a week after all signs of infection have disappeared.

What is ringworm?
Another fungal skin condition, ringworm is highly contagious. However, it is a bit of a misnomer, since there is no worm as such involved. What happens is that you develop

a ring shape of raised sore pink skin – a bit like a weal – in areas of the body that are warm and moist: for instance, the groin, armpits, under the breasts and also the feet.

What causes ringworm?
Ringworm can sometimes be contracted from family pets – like cats and dogs, so you should check out your moggy and fido with the local vet, in order to avoid reinfection.

Ringworm: how you can help yourself
• The same treatments apply for ringworm as for athlete's foot: using creams like Canesten twice daily, though you should tell your chemist that it is ringworm you've got, in order for the appropriate anti-fungal product to be recommended.
• Ringworm of the groin is very common in people who play sports – it can be spread by sharing a towel, so avoid this. Hygiene is important.
• Wash your clothes regularly and separately from the family's.
• Raise your general health through better eating habits (see Chapter 7).
• Some people find crushed or sliced garlic applied locally to the ringworm and bandaged in place really helps. It may sound very odd – but garlic is a potent anti-fungal agent. Renew twice daily – and it will also help you to avoid vampires!

NAPPY RASH

Another common skin condition which, as its name suggests, affects babies. Nearly all babies get red and sore bottoms from time to time – however well you keep them clean, so if your little one is currently suffering from a painful bot, don't give yourself a hard time about being a bad mum!

What causes nappy rash?

If you think about it, a tender baby's bottom is in constant contact with faeces and urine for around two years of its life, so it's small wonder that sometimes that supersoft skin will break out with a rash or a few spots. Diarrhoea can trigger nappy rash, as can urine soaking a nappy until it chafes. This, combined with an infection from the yeast, candida, leads to contamination of the skin, and sometimes this can spread beyond the nappy area to the abdomen.

Nappy rash: how you can help baby

• It goes without saying that you should keep your baby's bottom as clean as possible, and change nappies at regular intervals.

• Make sure baby's bottom is dry – especially around the skin creases.

• Try and 'air' his or her bottom as much as possible – obviously at the risk of a few minor accidents!

• Anti-fungal creams can be bought especially for this condition – Sudocrem, Kamillosan Baby Cream and Boots Nappy Rash Cream are all excellent.

• To help protect your baby's skin from continuous exposure to moisture, use a barrier cream, for example, zinc and castor oil. All these products are quite safe.

• If your baby wears terry towelling nappies, make sure to sterilise them while the infection is present. And ensure that all detergent is thoroughly rinsed out, as this too can trigger nappy rash.

• A good homeopathic product that can help nappy rash is calendula cream.

CHAPTER 4

Dry and Inflamed Skin Conditions

ECZEMA, DERMATITIS AND PROBLEM DRY SKIN

Eczema, and the umbrella term dermatitis, are all about the skin becoming inflamed. And when skin becomes inflamed, it is usually accompanied by a maddening urge to scratch. Inflamed skin conditions affect more than one in ten people. So rest assured, though you may feel scabby, scratchy, scaly and singled out – you're definitely not alone!

In the past, people used to distinguish between eczema and dermatitis. It was generally held that eczema was an inflammation of the skin caused by goings-on within the body, and that dermatitis was an inflammation caused by external forces. However, nowadays, dermatologists tend to think that the differences aren't quite so clear cut, and most now use the terms eczema and dermatitis interchangeably.

The word eczema comes from ancient Greece – and literally means 'to boil over'; given this is sometimes exactly how you feel when suffering from eczema, it's a pretty appropriate name!

Lucy's story
Looking at Lucy today, it is hard to believe she once suffered a terrible attack of eczema. Her skin is clear, there is a

25

positive glow to her complexion, and not a spot in sight.

'Fifteen years ago, I was plagued by eczema. It started slowly – appearing in patches on the back of my legs for example, and on my hands – and it started to cover more and more of me. I tried everything. I went to my doctor, to a dermatologist – all to no avail. I tried everything they asked me to try. I hated having to cover myself in those creams *before* getting into a bath – frequently I was in floods of tears. I never thought I would find a cure, and then one day, a friend recommended Traditional Chinese Medicine. I was very sceptical, but I liked the way so much time was spent with me, finding out about me as well as my skin problem. I took all the disgusting herbal teas he recommended and miracle of miracles, they worked! I would recommend looking into alternative medicine for anyone who finds conventional medicine doesn't work.'

What does eczema look like?
Eczematous skin has a surface that looks white and flaky. This is because the skin is producing less of the natural sebum which keeps the dead skin cells stuck together – so the scales are shed more frequently – hence the flakes. If the skin is scratched a lot, the outer layer of dead cells can become cracked, thus allowing germs to pass more easily into the skin. The skin gets infected and the outer layer thickens and becomes scaly. One type causes itchy water blisters to appear on the surface which often weep and form a crust.

Problem dry skin tends to be less severe than either eczema or dermatitis, and is often caused by exposure to harsh weather, wearing certain clothes and washing – all of which can remove the oil from the surface of the skin, leaving it dry.

There are many different types of eczema and dermatitis that can affect you at any age: the following list tells you about the most common types and how to identify them.

SOME OF THE DIFFERENT TYPES OF ECZEMA AND DERMATITIS

Irritant Contact Dermatitis
Affecting: all age groups
Caused by: contact with irritants, like washing powders and chemicals
Symptoms: red, scaly and itchy dry skin

Allergic Contact Dermatitis
Affecting: mostly women
Caused by: sufferer becoming allergic to substances like nickel** in cheap jewellery, rubber and elastic, some plants, some cooking utensils and also perfumes
Symptoms: can affect any part of the body; leaves skin red, scaly, itchy and dry

Atopic Eczema
Affecting: all age groups – especially children
Caused by: family genes – associated with asthma and hay fever, and often made worse by pets, house and dust mites
Symptoms: red scaly skin, sometimes forms a crust that can be itchy and painful; affects whole body, particularly the inside of wrists, elbows and back of knees

Seborrhoeic Eczema

Affecting: babies and adults, most common among men

Caused by: not known, but a type of yeast may in part cause this condition

Symptoms: can give skin a reddish tone; often affects scalp, and folds in body; usually clears up on its own

Discoid Eczema

Affecting: adults

Caused by: unknown

Symptoms: coin-shaped patches of eczema; affects those with dry skin

Asteatotic Eczema

Affecting: older people with dry skin

Caused by: lack of moisture

Symptoms: makes skin look like crazy paving

** Negotiations are currently taking place in the European Parliament which hopefully will lead to a ban on nickel in costume jewellery. Information sheets on contact dermatitis and nickel allergy are available from the National Eczema Society (see Useful Addresses).

Eczema and viral infections

Surprisingly, the common **cold sore** which we discussed in Chapter 2 can become a serious problem for anyone with **atopic eczema**. Atopic eczema sufferers do not develop normal immunity, and if they come into contact with someone suffering from a cold sore, it can lead to widespread infection, with the virus covering the whole skin surface. It is therefore essential that you steer clear of anyone with a cold sore, and particularly in the case of small children and babies, make sure that they don't come into contact with the cold sore virus. It is tempting for a mum with a cold sore to kiss and cuddle her baby – but you will just have to resist until the infection clears. Prompt treatment works and leaves no scarring, but it is much better to prevent than cure.

Can eczema be cured?
Though it is hard, there are a number of ways you can combat this condition, as Lucy's happy story reveals. We discuss Traditional Chinese Medicine in Chapter 9 – others have found homeopathy works wonders (see Chapter 11). Eczema is a complex subject and there are numerous specialist books you can consult to identify your own particular brand, but in any case, if you think you have eczema, you should see your doctor first and he or she will help you find out which type you've got, and which treatment might suit you best. But don't give up if one course of treatment doesn't seem to be working for you. Some people swear by Traditional Chinese Medicine while others find relief through homeopathy alone.

Problem dry skin often can disappear with the correct use of special emollients (see below).

Eczema: how you can help yourself
Do try considering:

- Traditional Chinese Medicine (TCM)
- Homeopathy
- Evening Primrose Oil
- Herbal remedies (see Chapter 10)
- Looking at your diet: a food supplement like spirulina may help

- Changing your home environment (see Chapter 15)
- Wearing cotton clothes
- Wearing rubber gloves when you wash up (except if you have **allergic contact dermatitis** and rubber affects you)
- Contacting the National Eczema Society (see Useful Addresses)
- Preserving the moisture content of your skin. Use the emollients and bath preparations listed below.

Some emollients that are popular with sufferers
Bath E45
Boots Calamine and Glycerin Cream
Boots Hydrocortisone Ointment
Dermidex
Lanacane
Psoriderm
Savlon
Wash E45/Cream E45
Unguentum Merck Cream
Balneum and Balneum Plus Bath treatments
See also Chapter 13.

Avoid
- Stressful situations
- Scratching – of course!
- Harshly and highly perfumed soap or bath additives
- Too-hot water in your bath; take showers or short, cool baths
- Wearing wool, or woollen mixtures

PSORIASIS

Remember Michael Gambon playing the hospital patient in Dennis Potter's television drama, *The Singing Detective*? If you're not sure exactly what psoriasis is, then this unforgettable image of suffering should help. Having said that, the main character was afflicted with a really debilitating form of psoriasis, and though the drama helped raise public awareness of the condition, it has also left many people with the impression that psoriasis is always chronic. Not so! There are plenty of psoriatics out there with relatively mild symptoms!

What is psoriasis?
In simple terms, psoriasis is just a vast acceleration of the usual replacement processes of the skin. Normally, a skin cell matures in twenty-one to forty days, and at the skin's surface, a continual shedding of dead cells, as scales, takes place. Psoriatic cells speed up the turnover process to just two to three days, and in such chaotic profusion (one thousand times faster than normal) that even live cells reach the surface and join forces with the dead ones in visible layers.

When scraped or scratched, these patches of cells show fine silvery scales. Mostly, they appear on key areas of the body, like the knees, elbows and scalp, though unfortunately for the sufferer, the face too can often be affected. And in extreme cases, as with the lead character in *The Singing Detective* – and indeed, Dennis Potter himself – psoriasis can affect the whole body. Potter suffered from crippling psoriatic arthropathy, which is a form of psoriasis linked with chronic arthritis.

Psoriasis is an upsetting condition, because not only do

you have to contend with discomfort, and a desperate desire
to scratch your way to relief no matter whether that scratching will make the condition worse or not, you also understandably feel very self-conscious indeed – especially if those
unsightly patches are prominent on the face. In many ways,
the psychological and social effects of this condition, far
outweigh the physical.

What causes psoriasis?
A number of things can trigger a first attack of psoriasis. A
throat infection, some drug treatments, burns, sunburn,
picking at another skin injury – even a stressful life event
like the death of a loved one, or marital problems, can
precipitate this skin condition. Stress can often lead to skin
flare ups generally.

Is it infectious?
Though unpleasant to look at, let me stress that in no way is
psoriasis infectious. It cannot be passed on from one person
to another by contact – and you can confidently correct
anyone who fears catching it from you. It can be very hurtful
to have people shy away from you, just because your skin is
patchy – so don't be afraid to speak out! Often, all people
want is reassurance; give it and you will both feel more at
ease, and chances are you'll win admiration for not beating
about the bush.

Who gets psoriasis?
Psoriasis affects approximately 80 million people worldwide,
and 1.5 million people in Britain alone – that's at least one in
fifty people fated with a condition that leaves inflamed and
scaly patches on the skin.
   Psoriasis affects both men and women equally. It can

appear for the first time at any age, although most sufferers first experience symptoms between the ages of ten and forty-five, and often at puberty or during the late teens. For the poor adolescent sufferer who is concerned enough with the problems of looking good and feeling cool, this must seem like fate is playing a very dirty trick! At the same time, some women sufferers have found that psoriasis is less prevalent during pregnancy whilst others have reported the start of symptoms around the time of the menopause, all of which could suggest that hormones are running amok in some form.

There is also a tendency for psoriasis to run in families, with about 30% of sufferers having relatives who also have psoriasis. However, though the chances are increased, rest assured it does not necessarily follow that just because Uncle Bert's got the scratchy patches, your newborn babe will follow suit! Also, people who suffer from inflammatory diseases like arthritis tend to have a greater tendency towards psoriasis.

Can psoriasis be cured?
Unfortunately not; it can only be kept at bay. Treatments today aim at reducing inflammation and controlling the rate of cell division. Cells in affected areas multiply excessively faster than the normal rate, producing layer upon layer of flaking dead skin.

Ultraviolet light or PUVA treatment as it is known, can help. It means ultraviolet light (UVA) combined with some pills called psoralens – hence PUVA. The pills are taken two hours before exposure to UVA and the treatment is repeated two to three times a week. We go into PUVA in more detail in Chapter 6. Some sufferers don't always enjoy the process. As one lady put it: 'I had to stand

33

completely naked in something that looked like Doctor Who's Tardis, and wearing sunglasses too. It's a long-winded process – you build up to sessions lasting an hour at a stretch, and you end up with a deep tan, which isn't so fashionable these days!'

Gentle sunbathing is also beneficial – though in the light of so much bad press, this should be taken very gently indeed. Also, the Dead Sea, as we shall see in Chapter 13, is a haven for skin sufferers since the minerals, sunshine, mud and salt water all seem to play a part in helping to clear the condition. There is even an International Psoriasis Treatment Centre there.

If all this sounds too expensive, hope could be in sight in the near future, if current tests in the UK for a new drug treatment prove successful. The drug, glucosaminyl muramyl dipeptide or, to make life easier, GMDP, was first tested in Russia last year – and all but two of twenty-four sufferers reported an improvement in their condition. Unlike other drugs now in use, GMDP seems to be free of serious side-effects.

Psoriasis: how you can help yourself

• Some sufferers have found that visualising the skin becoming clearer, for ten minutes each day while relaxing, has proved tremendously helpful.

• One woman found an old wives' remedy really helped her. She drank two cups of cooled boiled water daily. After a few weeks, the psoriasis started to disappear. Sounds cranky, but maybe worth a go.

• Try joining the Psoriasis Association where you can be assured of mutual support from fellow sufferers. (See Useful Addresses at the back of the book.)

Also:

- Light therapy (see Chapter 6)
- Relaxation
- Homeopathic remedies
- Herbal tinctures
- Including oily fish in your diet, or fish oil supplements

Lotions, potions and emollients
- Dead Sea bath salts
- Balneum Plus
- E45 dermatological skin care
- Petroleum jelly
- Psoriderm bath emulsion
- Aveeno range of cleansers (derived from refined oatmeal, which cleanses by absorbing grease and dirt from surface of skin)
- Coal tar (messy but effective)
- Salicylic acid (used to soften and lift off scales from the surface of the skin; a shampoo containing salicylic acid is often prescribed for loosening thick scales on the scalp and will need to be used on a daily basis for two to three weeks)
- Medicated shampoo like Meted, Pentrax and Capasal
- Aloe vera, applied topically or taken internally
- Vitamin D ointments and creams – these are the newest of self-help treatments for psoriasis and are proving very effective. They are odourless, easy to use and stain-free. Use the treatments twice daily until the skin is clear. These preparations are not currently recommended for the face.

See also Chapter 13.

Avoid
• Getting stressed out. This can cause a flare up, so learn to relax! Take up yoga, learn how to meditate or practise simple breathing techniques.
• Scratching, if you possibly can help it. Yes, yes, I know – that sort of comment when you're in the throes of a really itchy session can be extremely irritating! But better than scratching, try soothing your skin with a suitable emollient (see Chapter 13 for more details).
• Using soaps and detergents which can be extra irritants, causing unnecessary and excessive dryness. In the bath, use a moisturising soap substitute – again, our section on bathing in Chapter 13 will help you here.

SCABIES

An extraordinary story appeared in the *New Scientist* a few months ago: 'Musicians at the San Francisco Opera are suffering an epidemic of scabies – with at least one cellist itching so badly she had to put her bow down for a scratch mid-performance. The outbreak is puzzling public health officials because scabies mites, which cause the furious itching when they burrow under the skin, do not usually spread by casual contact. The opera house, meanwhile, has been fumigated from top to bottom.'

Oddball as this little tale is, it goes to illustrate how quickly a skin condition like scabies can spread. Not surprisingly, it is popularly known just as 'itch'.

What is scabies?
Like head lice, the scabies mites live in or on the skin. Female scabies mites, only just visible to the eye, burrow

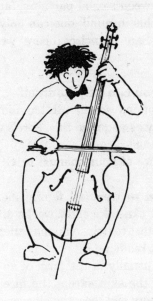

under the skin and lay their eggs near the surface. The eggs hatch in three or four days, and become adults in ten to fourteen days. Intense itching and irritation are the first sign of infection and the sufferer begins to scratch which in turn brings on a rash – usually between the fingers, around the wrists, the feet, the genital region and elbows; rarely are the face and neck infected. The more you scratch that rash, the more the skin will appear scaly, red and blistery.

What causes scabies?
Scabies can affect anyone, regardless of how meticulous they might be about personal hygiene. The mites are spread by

direct contact as opposed to casual – hence their propensity to be passed between sexual partners, family members and children. With this in mind, one can only imagine that the players in the San Francisco opera were a pretty close bunch!

Scabies: how you can help yourself
If these descriptions sound all too familiar, and you're itching like crazy as you read this, here's what to do:

● Seek the advice of your chemist or GP to establish it is indeed scabies.
● You will need to treat all family members as well as yourself, since it can take eight weeks after the first infection before you start to itch – you may therefore have spread the mite without realising it.
● Treatment is usually in the form of an insecticide lotion, applied to all of the skin except the face. Pay attention to between the fingers and toes, the elbows, genital region and palms of the hands. Your chemist will advise which lotion is best, though water-based ones are preferable to those containing alcohol, since they are gentler on the skin and less likely to sting.
● As long as you apply the lotion correctly, you need only treat your body once, and you don't need to bathe beforehand.
● You may continue to itch after the treatment, sometimes for several weeks, but only repeat the treatment if there is still evidence of the presence of mites. Calamine lotion should soothe the itching in the meantime.
● Don't scrub away at your skin – this won't remove the mites and will only exacerbate the irritation.

TO SCRATCH, OR NOT TO SCRATCH

Sue's story

'I had eczema in my teens – now thankfully all but gone, with the help of TCM and homeopathy. What I'll never forget, though, is the hell I went through wanting to scratch the whole time. Sometimes, it got so bad, I'd take a plastic hairbrush to it, and savagely attack the spot where it itched the most. Of course that only made matters worse, and my skin would weep – but at the time, it was like the sweetest most satisfying sensation you can imagine!

'In the end, I got help from a medical psychologist, who trained me out of the itch-scratch-itch cycle. I'm sure if that hadn't have happened, my skin would have taken that much longer to heal.'

Sounds familiar? The bliss of answering the persistent call of an itch . . . Everyone relates to that, even those blessed beings who don't have an on-going skin problem. I was once bitten so badly by mosquitoes while camping in Italy that, like Sue, I was attacking the soles of my feet with a hairbrush – I did of course clean it before using it on my hair! I also totally relate to that sense of relief, albeit a temporary one, that a good scratching can bring.

Suffice to say, scratching won't do you any good at all, despite what that devil sitting on your shoulder tells you. Scratching an itch seems such an automatic thing to do – but let's face it, it makes skin raw, sometimes infected, often thick and leathery too. And most importantly, it can stop the healing process. If sore skin is left alone, it will heal itself – providing there is no infection. But if you scratch it, you set the healing process back a step or two.

Remember, though you cannot turn off an itch, you don't have to scratch it.

Breaking the itch-scratch-itch cycle

Sue talked about her success in breaking the itch-scratch-itch cycle – and though it may sound impossible when you're in the throes of an itching frenzy, you *can* block the response to scratch. The first step is to treat your skin problem with the correct emollients on a regular basis. Then, whenever your skin feels uncomfortable, top up with more cooling emollient, used thinly and applied gently. Take antihistamines if they help.

If you do feel the urge to scratch, try diverting your thoughts on to something else, and chances are, the itch will stop eventually. It's a bit like breaking the smoking habit.

Another good trick: pinch the area you want to scratch. Or press a fingernail into it. You could try putting something cold onto the itch, like a bag of frozen peas, or some ice cubes – that will soon stop the feverish urge.

When do you most want to scratch? Is it last thing at night, for example? I know that when I had **irritant dermatitis** on my legs, the itching got worse when I removed my socks or stockings before going to bed. Make sure you have fully rinsed your socks and stockings after washing them. I once noticed that my black socks still bore the traces of soap powder from the washing machine, a surefire way to kick off an itch! If, like me, your itching gets worse when you're undressing, try to speed up the process. Do something else at the same time, like talking to somebody (a partner, family member or good friend, naturally – your neighbour may find your request for help in undressing rather odd!) Don't think about scratching – listen to some music, or a radio programme instead. Some people find a bath helps, providing it's not too hot.

Also, there are certain skin care products designed to help you with bathing, which we'll talk about further in

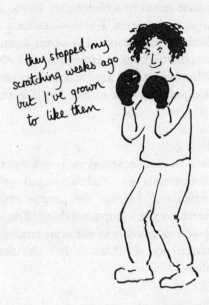

they stopped my scratching weeks ago but I've grown to like them

Chapter 13. An example is Balneum Plus bath treatment, which you can buy from Boots, and which actually treats your skin while you bathe. Also, it contains a special ingredient which relieves itching fast. It soothes and softens the affected area for up to seven hours, and is said to protect against further itching – so this might be ideal for your night-time dip.

Keep your nails cut short and blunt – so that if the urge gets too much, at least there won't be any sharp edges to do more damage to your skin. Keep the bedroom cool, because an overhot environment will only make you want to scratch even more. Also, drinking alcohol heats the body up, and that too will make you itchy – so remember, moderation at all times!

Microscopic dust mites can really play havoc with people suffering from skin problems. But maintaining a dust-free environment sounds impossible, I'll admit – unless you're chronically houseproud like Hyacinth in *Keeping Up Appearances*. However, there are manageable steps you can take towards keeping the dust at bay. We'll discuss these in Chapter 15.

Habit reversal
Sue sought help from a hospital in breaking her itching habit. Several hospitals run habit-reversal programmes, which are particularly helpful for people with **chronic eczema** who find they can't stop scratching. Your doctor will be able to tell you if your local hospital runs such a programme. Alternatively, ask him or her to refer you to a clinical psychologist.

CHAPTER 5

Acne and its Mimics

ACNE

Peter's story

'I got acne at around the age of thirteen, and really it lasted all through my teens, and well into my twenties. My brother had it too. I had the lot – whiteheads, blackheads, even boils! It made me feel quite unlike anyone else – ugly, a total outcast in fact, not that anyone teased me specifically. With girls, it became a major factor, in that I was far too shy to try and ask them out.

'I became the world's greatest expert at picking my spots – sorry to be so revolting! I would pick them until they bled, and now of course, I've got pock marks to show for it. Apart from that major sin, I treated the acne as best I knew how in those days. I washed regularly with soap and water, and used an ointment called Escamol which was popular at the time. It all helped in a minor way, but the acne never disappeared completely.

'Yes, I did seek medical help, but the doctor was neither very enlightening nor sympathetic as such. He just told me to carry on washing properly, and using the ointment. No one asked me about diet, which was typical of a schoolboy's then: loads of fried food, no fresh fruit and very little in the way of properly cooked vegetables. I'm now fifty-two, and I still get the odd pimple – particularly when I'm under stress.'

Peter's tale must ring bells for many poor sufferers plagued by teenage spots and pimples. In fact, though people think of acne as a teenage problem (some 70% of teenagers suffer acne in one form or another), there are plenty of us who sail through our teens and twenties with perfectly clear skin, only to wake up at thirty plus with an uncalled for covering of zits! And if you are one of the 5% of women and 1% of men over the age of forty who still has significant problems with acne, rest assured, you are not alone – and treatment is available.

Acne, therefore, is a common enough skin condition, but it can leave big psychological scars as well as small 'physical' ones. But help is at hand – people get over acne, and even when it seems at its worst, there are plenty of things you can do to help yourself.

The myths
Let's get these out of the way right from the start:
Acne is not caused by dirt.
Acne is not caused by eating too many fry-ups.
Acne is not caused by making a pig of yourself with chocolate.
Acne is not caused by too much/not enough sex.

So what does cause acne?
This inflammatory skin condition runs in families, and can range from mild, where the face is covered by just a few spots, to severe – and it can affect the skin on the face, neck, back and chest. Acne is related to hormonal imbalance; that's why it attacks so many young people, boys especially, at a time when the body is in a state of such dramatic change and flux.

Potential triggers of acne

Over-production of oil
In 'calm' skin, the fatty substance known as sebum, which is produced by the sebaceous glands attached to the tiny hairs covering the skin, acts as a natural 'oil' or lubricant. But, around the time of puberty, too much of this sebum tends to get produced – triggered particularly by male sex hormones which control the sebaceous glands. These hormones are called androgens – the main androgen is that celebrated stuff called testosterone, a hormone which through name and image has inspired everything from aftershave to Italian fast cars! Well, both sexes have testosterone in their blood, though admittedly, men have around five times more of the stuff than women do. Girl acne sufferers apparently have slightly greater levels of male sex hormones in their blood than other girls of their age – and although this by no means indicates a lack of femininity on their part, it is probably a factor in making them more susceptible to acne. Interestingly, eunuchs have very little testosterone, they secrete hardly any sebum, and consequently you don't find many eunuchs with acne.

Exercise
Around 15% of sufferers find that their acne flares up when they've been sweating a lot. This is probably because water swells up the hair duct even further, so that there is a complete blockage which, in turn, leads to inflammation. OK, all you couch potatoes, this might seem like a heaven-sent excuse to stop exercising – but exercise can really benefit the skin as it boosts the skin's function and helps eliminate circulation problems. The answer is to wear light absorbent clothing, and to make sure that you work out in

an aerated space. If you tend to sweat anyway, regardless of exertion, then think about wearing natural clothing rather than synthetic materials. For certain skin conditions like **eczema**, it is extremely important to wear cottons and other natural fibres.

Your environment

The same goes for your environment. If you work in a kitchen, say, or steamy room, this can make your acne flare up. So too a holiday, for those lucky enough to be travelling somewhere exotic in the tropics, where the weather, if steamy and muggy, can exacerbate the problem. Try to keep the skin clean and pat the sweat off with a hygienic wipe.

Periods and the pill

Some women find they develop spots just before their monthly periods – for some, it is a surefire indication that their periods are about to begin – again, this would indicate a hormonal link. The contraceptive pill can improve acne in some cases, whereas the condition can make an unwelcome first appearance around the time of the menopause.

Stress

As Peter's story indicates, stress and anxiety can also contribute to the problem. But don't despair. Stick with the self-help suggestions we recommend, and you should be delighted by the change in your skin.

What happens in an acne attack

Blockage of the hair duct

The pore or duct, through which hairs emerge, begins to be blocked by 'sticky' dead skin cells lining the duct. In normal skin, these cells continually grow and die, and are shed into the duct and up onto the surface of the skin. In acne sufferers, the cells react abnormally, and instead of being shed, they progressively block the duct. It's a bit like a kettle getting furred up. With the duct blocked, sebum flow is obstructed, and the oil solidifies, and eventually darkens because it contains melanin. This is a blackhead. If the opening becomes blocked completely, the sebaceous gland will enlarge, and a whitehead is formed.

Actually, the story of why blackheads are called blackheads is rather amusing. In the dark old days when microscopes were thin on the ground, it was widely believed that blackheads were tiny worms living in the skin – and that the black bit was the head of the worm. No wonder the myth exists that acne is caused by dirt!

Inflammation
Inflammation and pus formation are also thought to be caused by an acute build up of oil. Once the pore is blocked, oil collects around the hair and hair root, and this becomes infected with a particular bacterium which usually lives harmlessly on your skin. This triggers off the body's defence mechanism, and white blood cells start to battle with the bacteria just beneath the skin. The result? A papule when the skin is inflamed, which, if a yellow head forms, becomes a pustule or zit – two charming names for what is a charmless red spot with a yellow head.

The unwanted, unloved zit can grow still further into a painful inflamed cyst in severe cases of acne. This happens when the walls of the duct and sebaceous gland rupture under the skin surface. Cysts are several times larger than an ordinary papule or pustule, and are most commonly found on the back, the back of the neck, the shoulders, the jawline

47

and chest. Eventually they will disappear, but they are more likely to leave scars than ordinary spots.

To squeeze or not to squeeze

In the natural evolution of that zit, pus eventually ruptures onto the surface of the skin and the zit will settle down. But, forgive the pun, let's face it – how many of you are disciplined enough to let evolution have its own way? The temptation to squeeze early on in the life of that zit can be huge. Sometimes, you can get into a mad self-destructive cycle with squeezing. You know logically it will make your skin worse, but you feel pretty hideous anyway so 'Who cares?' you say to yourself, and away go those nails, burrowing into the flesh. Also, there is something oddly satisfying about emptying a zit of its nasty contents – everyone secretly knows this, though few will admit it! Perhaps someone should do a study on the pleasures of zit popping . . . but I digress. Take it from the experts, if you give way to the temptation to squeeze, the pus may rupture *into* the skin, which will cause even greater inflammation and possibly scarring too. Remember, if in doubt, don't, and if you do and you squeeze until you see blood, you're on the way to possible scars.

Some women (and it does tend to be more a woman's habit than a man's) pick at really quite minor pimples to the extent that the head of the spot forms a scab and looks quite raw. Picking is a very common habit, but people who attack minor spots repeatedly tend to be obsessive, anxious types – and often a little supportive counselling can be as helpful as any lotion or potion.

Scarring

Scarring often occurs with acne, and can be very severe. About a fifth of sufferers have some degree of scarring. This ranges from visible pit holes commonly known as pock marks, where a hair follicle has become infected and inflamed and is unable to regain its original shape, to hypertrophic scars caused by cysts, which are pink, dome-shaped and hard to the touch, and will probably clear up in a few months, to keloid scars. These are scars which appear to have grown beyond the barriers of the inflamed spot or cyst. They are mostly found on the chest and over the shoulders.

Prevention of scarring is possible, as long as the acne is treated at an early stage. Bad keloid scars can last into middle or old age – but even then, will improve with time. You can ask your doctor about drug treatment for severe scarring, or you might want to consider collagen replacement therapy, plastic surgery or chemical peeling, all of which can help improve the appearance of the skin's surface. We will discuss some of these options in Chapter 14.

Should I avoid make-up?

Some beauty routines are well worth adopting, like a regular clay facial mask, or a facial steam which will help open pores and release impurities. These would suit both men and women, so don't be put off by that word 'beauty', all you guys! For women, avoid using compressed powder or loose powder which can block pores still further. If you want to camouflage the worst spots, use a non-greasy cosmetic base or a medicated blemish stick and cream. Certain hair oils, like those to defrizz very curly hair, can induce spots along the margin of the hair. These should be avoided. It is also important to remove your make-up carefully last thing at night. For beneficial beauty tips, see Chapters 13 and 14.

Should I avoid shaving?

The parts of your face where you need to shave the most also tend to be the areas where you get the most spots, and your skin feels most sensitive. If your spots are particularly bad, you should avoid shaving the affected areas until your skin is calmer.

Does diet affect acne?

Despite popular myth, there is no sure evidence that chocolate and fried foods make acne worse. In fact, American researchers have fed volunteers excessive amounts of chocolate in order to prove there is no link between the two. The volunteers may have felt a little queasy, but their spots remained the same! I'm not suggesting that this gives you free rein to go mad on Mars Bars – eating too many sweet things won't be the most healthy diet for anyone! Obviously, if some foods seem to make your spots worse, you should try and avoid them, and in any case, aim to eat a healthy balanced diet, and 'flush through' with lots of water. Our nutrition chapter will give you some helpful hints.

Is acne caused by dirt?

Obsessively cleaning your skin with one of the many advertised acne preparations won't improve your acne. In fact, acne is no more common on dirty skin than clean. Blackheads look dirty, which may have given rise to the myth, but as we saw, the black of a blackhead is caused by pigmentation, not dirt. Regular washing with a mild or medicated soap, twice a day, is all that is needed.

As acne sufferers have more than their fair share of natural oil production on their skin, bacteria can spread – especially in warm and muggy environments. In this case, antibacterial skin washes are useful.

Can it be cured?

Your doctor may prescribe antibiotics if your acne is severe. But there is still a place for over-the-counter creams and lotions. All sorts of acne treatments are currently bringing remarkable relief to countless sufferers, so don't 'wait until you grow out of it' – do something now. Don't let acne stop you getting on with your life! You will need to persevere for any of the treatments to be successful, however, often for months at a time. But do stick with it, the results are worth it.

Acne: how you can help yourself

• Try topical preparations like anti-bacterial skin-washing creams: Biactol, Clearasil, etc.

• Preparations containing salicylic acid or benzoyl peroxide which encourage drying and peeling of the skin's surface to help unblock the ducts and allow the sebum to flow. They are available in different strengths. Start with 2.5% and gradually build up both the time the treatment is left on the skin, and the concentration. It may take four to six weeks for benzoyl peroxide to take effect, so be patient. If your skin gets very red or feels irritated (blondes and redheads seem to be most at risk), talk to your chemist. To counteract the stinging side-effects of benzoyl peroxide, some preparations may contain hydrocortisone which calms the skin.

• Sulphur treatments, particularly effective for people with mild acne and for those who can't use benzoyl peroxide. Sulphur concentrations can kill bacteria and come in the form of lotions, potions, creams and gels. Improvements can often be seen after just a week, but be warned – the smell sulphur gives of rotting eggs can be very off-putting!

- Vitamin A derivatives like Retin-A also known as tretinoin, can help in the form of creams, gels or lotions, but can also cause sensitivity.

Also worth trying:

- A gentle exfoliating scrub can help once a week, but not if you are using benzoyl peroxide or if acne is inflamed.
- Many acne treatments work by drying out your skin. But even oily skin needs moisture – so look out for greaseless gels, or oil-free moisturisers which will soothe and calm the skin. Be gentle with your skin and avoid harsh products.
- Some people find taking a beta-carotene and zinc supplement helps them.
- Shampooing your hair regularly and keeping it off your face is a good idea.
- Eat plenty of fresh fruit and vegetables.
- Sunshine can help – in moderation. It dries out spots for some people. Use a non-greasy gel sun protector, rather than an oil.
- Homeopathic remedies like Belladonna and Pulsatilla may help.
- Tea tree oil, available from the Body Shop.
- Herbal remedies like Soothene Ointment.
- Aromatherapy is thought to be of help to acne sufferers. We will talk more about this in Chapter 13.

ROSACEA

Some skin disorders mimic acne, but are actually quite different and need a different form of treatment. Rosacea, also known by the misnomer, acne rosacea, is one of these.

What is rosacea?

It is a relatively common long-term skin problem, particularly with middle-aged people, and its symptoms range from repeated blushing attacks, progressing through to permanent red skin with a smattering of broken veins, to acne-like pustules and lumps.

Some facts about rosacea

• The skin around the cheeks, forehead, chin and nose appears very red and inflamed, rather similar in appearance to a rash, and has little thread-like veins running over it.

• Sufferers usually have less greasy skin than in cases of true acne.

• Rosacea is not a life-threatening condition – though, because it affects your appearance, it can cause undue distress.

• Occasionally the skin will become inflamed elsewhere, for instance on the chest or back.

• Rosacea is not infectious: it can't be caught or passed on to any one else.

• Modern drugs can be very effective in curing rosacea.

• Menopausal flushing can make rosacea worse – ask your GP about medicines to control the flushing.

What causes rosacea?

Nobody knows what causes rosacea exactly – but the common understanding is that this condition is due to a disorder of the tiny blood vessels which supply the skin. Sometimes, if you have been overusing a steroid cream to treat other skin conditions on the face, you can develop rosacea, because the blood vessels on the face have become damaged.

Who gets rosacea?

Rosacea tends to run in families, and many people mistake the typical florid complexion of a sufferer for a family characteristic which has to be 'lived with' rather than treated – although rosacea responds well to treatment. Rosacea tends to affect more women than men – and often it is middle-aged women who suffer the most. Indeed, one in ten women aged between thirty and fifty-five may suffer from mild rosacea. Having said that, if men get rosacea, they tend to get far worse attacks, often leading to rhinophyma. This is when the tip of the nose becomes purple-red and the skin over the nose thickens to become coarse and bumpy.

Rosacea can start during the teens – with occasional flushing on the face in situations where the sufferer is nervous, embarrassed or stressed. Alcohol and spicy foods can exacerbate the condition. If you are prone to rosacea, these flushing attacks can get worse during your twenties. Your skin will feel hot, and the attack will usually last only a few minutes, after which it will return to its normal state. In your thirties, pustules and papules can occur on the face – hence the confusion with acne. With more severe cases, rosacea can irritate the eyelids, causing eyes to get bloodshot – and the face may even swell up.

The true cause of rosacea is unknown – but skin type is relevant. The typical 'Celtic' fair skin is more prone than any other type.

Rosacea: how you can help yourself

First of all, visit your GP to establish that your condition is indeed rosacea, and not due to sun exposure, dermatitis or even alcoholic flushing. You may be referred to a dermatologist.

Rosacea tends to respond well to antibiotics, taken either orally or as a topical cream – more so than with general cases of acne. Antibiotic tablets can also help if you are one of the poor unfortunates whose eyes get irritated or bloodshot during an attack. Within a few days of taking a prescribed treatment, the papules and pustules should start to disappear, and further deterioration of the skin should be halted at this stage. If you think this is the route you want to pursue, then consult your GP. In any case, it might be worth consulting your GP – however mild your symptoms, since there are treatments available which will not only soothe and clear the skin, but will help prevent more serious problems developing later. Also, rosacea can flare up again despite sometimes several years' respite. As soon as the rash reappears, you should see your doctor promptly for more treatment.

In severe cases, where broken veins are very visible, a specialist may advise surgical laser treatment. Lasers are being used successfully in treating broken veins, and no scarring will occur. Another method commonly used is an electric current which destroys unwanted veins. This process is called electrodesiccation – and is carried out by inserting a fine needle or electrode into the blood vessel, and then passing a current through it.

Flare ups can also be kept to a minimum by making certain changes to your life-style. These include:

• Avoiding food and drink that is too hot or too cold.
• Keeping stressful situations to a minimum – and learning to relax.
• Steering clear of alcohol if that tends to make your flushing worse.
• Using oil-free cosmetic products and creams.

- Avoiding too much exposure to the sun.
- Avoiding caffeine – change to decaffeinated tea and coffee, and caffeine-free colas and drinks.
- Trying a wheat- and milk-free diet, vitamin supplements and skin-softening treatments.

Contact the Rosacea Information Line on 0891 517200 for more information.

HIVES/URTICARIA

Hives and urticaria are one and the same. Hives is the more common name but the condition is also known, confusingly, as nettle rash, because it is so similar to the skin eruptions caused by stinging nettles.

What are hives?
Hives is a skin condition triggered by an allergy. If the sufferer comes into contact with the substance to which he or she is allergic, either through contact, inhalation or ingestion, this will prompt certain cells in the body to release histamine, which in turn encourages blood vessels in the skin to become dilated. These vessels then leak fluid into the skin – hence the inflammation.

In general, the condition is identified by extremely itchy raised weals. These eruptions are generally pale in the centre, changing to red around the edges of the weal. They vary in size, from small pimple-like spots right through to bumpy patches spanning several inches. Sometimes blisters can form. They can be found in any number and on any part of the body – even on the lips and eyes.

Because the eruptions can appear rather suddenly and

56

dramatically on the surface of the skin, this can be scary if you don't know what is happening to you, but rest assured, these allergic attacks can be very short-lived, lasting from a few hours to a few days.

A more severe type of hives called angio-oedema occurs when the swellings are much more pronounced, and commonly affect the face, eyelids, arms, hands and throat. This strain can cause breathing difficulties and it is essential that you seek medical help immediately.

What causes hives?
The body is responding to the presence of a trigger substance by releasing histamine under the skin. The allergen which triggers an attack could be food, drugs, house dust, or animal skin flakes, as well as sensitivity to sunlight, pollen and the cold.

Some facts about causes of hives
• Stress can trigger hives as it has the effect of suppressing the body's immune system.
• It can be very difficult to track down the actual cause of an outbreak – for many people, it's a case of persistent detective work to try and find what triggers an attack.
• Common 'trigger' substances include: strawberries, shellfish, eggs, nuts, food preservatives and additives, artificial colourings and drugs like aspirin or antibiotics.
• Contact with certain substances can bring on an attack, for example, with certain cosmetics or insects. If breathing is affected, because of an insect sting for instance, you must get immediate help. Sometimes, just immersing your hands in cold water can cause weals to appear, as can contact with cold winds and rain.

Who gets hives?

Women can be particularly prone to this condition, especially where there is a hormonal imbalance present. Allergy-prone people tend to suffer from hives more frequently than others, so individuals who get hay fever, **eczema** and asthma can also be prone to hives. A tendency to hives can run in families.

Hives: how you can help yourself

The usual medical treatment for hives is to apply topical local anaesthetic products (look out for trade names like Caladryl and Lanacane) and anti-histamines like Triludan which are taken orally. All are readily available over the counter. However, it is always worth checking with your GP first.

In terms of helping yourself, if you suffer from hives regularly, you should:

● Avoid trigger foods like strawberries, nuts, shellfish and eggs (see the chapter on nutrition).
● Try and keep a food diary to help you eliminate the culprit ingredients.
● Avoid monosodium glutamate – the taste enhancer found in Chinese food. This is known to trigger attacks. Likewise the food colourant tartrazine, and flavourings like sali-cylates, used in ice creams, cake mixes, and soft drinks – and also found in seeds, dried fruits, thyme, dill, paprika and oregano.
● Be very careful about what cosmetics you use. Make sure they are hypo-allergenic.
● Are you currently taking penicillin – or the anti-inflammatory drugs commonly used for arthritic conditions? If so, check with your GP as these can sometimes trigger an attack.

• Consider homeopathic, vitamin and herbal treatments. Chlorelia, based on pure seaweed algae, is a good, easily absorbed supplement, and you could also try a natural anti-histamine called Histazyme, along with four grams of vitamin C each day.

• Pure aloe vera gel smoothed onto the hives will cool them down. A good health shop will stock this, or see Chapter 13 for more details.

• Chinese herbs are also known to help. To find your nearest TCM practitioner, send £1.50 plus SAE to the Register of Chinese Herbal Medicine, PO Box 400, Wembley, Middx HA9 9NE.

• Learn to combat stress in your life – many people find yoga to be of tremendous benefit.

CHAPTER 6

The Sun and Your Skin

Let's face it – many of us feel so sun starved, that at the merest hint of a fine day, we're out in the open, stripped to our birthday suits, and throwing caution to the wind.

OK, we have all become much more cautious about the hazards of unprotected sunbathing, but there are still plenty of fair-skinned people taking enormous risks in the sun. More and more Brits, for example, are escaping the winter gloom for the sunshine (some 500,000 go abroad over Christmas), but we are still not taking the threat of skin cancer seriously. After being cooped up in offices and homes for months on end, with our skin weak and unprepared, we then go completely mad for two weeks, and submit our poor pale bods to a fortnight's blast in the sunshine. Well, did you know that during those two weeks, it is possible to create as much damage to your skin as during the whole of the rest of the year spent in Britain? And the other mistake, that is easily made, is to assume that British sunshine isn't as harmful as the sunshine abroad, however hot it gets.

Some sunlight is in fact needed to help our bodies produce vitamin D – a vital vitamin for bone growth. Scientists reckon that around fifteen to twenty minutes' exposure to sunlight three times a week should produce sufficient amounts of vitamin D in order for the body to function healthily – but too much exposure to sunlight in the short term can lead to sunburn, and in the long term (i.e. repeated over-exposure), it can lead to premature wrinkles, and possible skin cancer.

Yet despite an ever increasing flood of publicity on the link between sun exposure and premature wrinkling, we are still conditioned into thinking that a tan looks great and healthy on anyone. Coco Chanel was the lady responsible for making Mediterranean tans so fashionable – all the more ironic then that sixty years on, the cosmetic companies are flogging outrageously expensive creams which blind us with scientific jargon, purporting to halt the damage to our sun-induced wrinkles! But in the same way that a hangover is nature's way of telling you you've overdone the alcohol, that glowing, seemingly healthy tan is actually your body's way of trying to protect the skin against damage. The cells of the skin go into over-drive to produce more of the protective pigment melanin. In dark-skinned people, there is plenty of this pigment – fair-skinned, redheads and freckled people have less and are therefore at greater risk of sunburn and skin cancer.

WHAT IS ULTRAVIOLET LIGHT?

Natural sunlight has three components; heat, visible light and ultraviolet radiation.

Ultraviolet radiation from the sun can be divided into various light waves, which are categorised according to their intensity. UVA rays have the longest wavelength, capable of penetrating the skin's deepest layer, where, at its most destructive, it can disturb the production of collagen and elastin – the 'bricks and mortar' of supple, youthful skin. UVA rays can also affect the epidermis, speeding up skin ageing, and are also pinpointed as the cause of sun rashes.

Although the shorter wavelength UVB rays only penetrate the skin's upper layer, or dermis, they are the main culprit in skin cancer. However, recent research suggests that the longer wave UVA rays are equally responsible for both burning and disease.

SUNBURN – WHAT HAPPENS AND HOW TO RECOGNISE IT

When skin cells get burnt by UVB rays, fluid leaks between them and sets off swelling. The affected area reddens as the capillaries dilate in an attempt to throw off excessive heat – hence the familiar lobster look of the Britisher abroad! Sunburn appears from around half an hour to several hours after exposure. In severe cases, swelling and blistering can occur, often getting worse on the second day, and sometimes accompanied by fever and a headache. Once the sunburn has settled down, the skin will begin to peel. The peeling is actually your body's way of getting rid of damaged skin cells.

Sunburn: how you can help yourself
Once you've been burnt, there is not an awful lot you can do to reverse the process – it is almost a case of having to grin and bear it. But there are some treatments you can employ to calm down the badly burnt skin:

• First and foremost, don't be tempted to burst blisters if

you have any – you risk attracting infection.
- A tepid bath can take the heat out of the burn.
- To soothe and calm, wrap the affected parts of the skin in water-soaked bandages.
- Stay out of the sun in a cool place – if you have to go out, cover your body completely with loose clothing.
- Make sure you drink plenty of liquids: preferably water and other non-alcoholic drinks. Part of the pain of sunburn is caused by loss of fluid in the burnt areas and alcohol will only dehydrate the body further.
- Calamine lotion and aloe vera gel will soothe burnt skin – apply liberally.
- Take painkillers if the skin is inflamed; aspirin actually has a specific ability to reduce sunburn inflammation, so use it in preference to other over-the-counter painkillers. If fever persists, see a doctor.

Prevention is better than cure . . .
Above all, try to avoid getting sunburnt. Here's how:

Identify your skin type first and foremost. Dermatologists divide the population into six different skin types – according to their response in the sun. Assess your type, then choose the correct sun protection factor in your suncreams.

Incidentally, there has been some considerable concern recently in the suncream industry, that many creams are only given sun protection factors according to how much protection they offer against UVB rays – with no guide to their effectiveness against the equally damaging UVA. However, this looks set to change in the near future – Boots the pharmacy chain, for example, have already introduced a UVA star rating system into their range, and other manufacturers will undoubtedly follow suit.

The skin types

Type 1: Always burns, never tans – generally fair-skinned with blue or green eyes and freckles. Use SPF 25–20.

Type 2: Can burn at first – then tans slowly with difficulty. Generally fair-haired and fair-skinned types. Use SPF 20–15.

Type 3: Tans slowly but easily, rarely burns, and if so, moderately: medium skin tone, light brown hair, blue, green or brown eyes. Use SPF 15.

Type 4: Tans easily, rarely burns – rare in the UK but common in Mediterranean countries: olive skin and brown eyes. Use SPF 15–8.

Type 5: Tans well, hardly ever burns: Indian or similar shade of brown skin. Use SPF 8.

Type 6: Never burns. Black, Afrocaribbean skin. Use SPF 6.

Shun the sun

Our skin types don't change, so there is no use hoping you will build up a resistance to the sun *and* stay healthy. Our skin has a sort of 'memory' – and the effect of over-exposure to the sun is both permanent and cumulative. Every time you take a two-week holiday in the sunshine, your skin is clocking up the memory in your epidermal cells. After fifty-odd years of playing lobster on the beach, the effect, not least in terms of wrinkles and loss of elasticity, is obvious. Remember, it is never too late to jump out of the lobster pot!!

If you have skin types 1 and 2, you will never achieve a safe deep golden tan, and any attempt to do so will very likely end in damage. If you insist on sunbathing, you should avoid the middle of the day when the sun is at its strongest – for example between 11 a.m. and 3 p.m. in the UK and between 12 and 4 p.m. in the Mediterranean. You should use a fairly high SPF sunscreen which must be reapplied every hour and a half, and always after swimming or exercise – even if the cream claims to be waterproof! However, repeated application of a high SPF cream doesn't mean you can stay out in the sun longer. Once you've had your maximum dose of sun, you should head for the shade. At the same time, you needn't get paranoid and smother yourself in SPF 60 as some Americans are now wont to do. Far better to enjoy a couple of hours of sun with a covering of SPF 15, than a whole day looking like a bleached as opposed to beached whale in SPF 60 plus! To calculate how long you can stay out in the sun, multiply the SPF by the time it takes you to burn when your skin is unprotected. For example, if you burn after ten minutes, using an SPF of 10 will mean you can stay safely exposed for 100 minutes.

Wear a hat to protect the hair and head, and drink plenty of water. Always wear good sunglasses which will protect your eyes from ultraviolet light – they will care not only for your eyes, but also the delicate skin around the eyes which is very prone to wrinkles! After being out in the sun, use plenty of moisturisers and for a week or two after returning home. Remember, too, that the skin of young children is very susceptible to skin damage and needs high protection. The Australian slogan: 'Kids Cook Quick' is basic, but to the point. Babies should not be exposed to the sun at all.

SUN RASHES

Sun rashes are quite common, and can be distinguished as sun-related, because the rash rarely occurs in places where the sun cannot reach, for example, under the chin, behind the ears, under the nose, etc. Essentially a blistery, sometimes itchy rash of this sort indicates that you are photosensitive, and no, that doesn't mean you dislike having your picture taken – but your body doesn't react very well to the sun and you are in effect allergic to it! You should always wear a high protection sunscreen and keep out of the sun as much as possible. If your skin develops a rash, calamine lotion or aloe vera gel are extremely soothing.

VITILIGO

More than half a million people in the UK suffer from this benign albeit psychologically upsetting, skin condition.

What is vitiligo?
This is a condition where patches of skin lose colour or pigment, and consequently become extremely sensitive to sun exposure. The patches are white in colour, and obviously extremely noticeable on darker skins. The most commonly affected areas are the face, armpits, hands and groin, and the patches tend to enlarge slowly over a number of months.

In around 30% of cases, the skin will regain its pigment. Where this happens, small brown spots will appear around the hair follicles. These will gradually spread and may coalesce to cover the white patch completely.

Vitiligo is not painful, infectious or life-threatening.

What causes vitiligo?
Nobody knows what triggers an attack of vitiligo, but it is often thought to be an auto-immune disorder – and one that starts in teenage years (sometimes earlier). It can run in families.

Vitiligo: how you can help yourself
- Use a good sunblocking cream to stop the white patches burning in the sun.
- Investigate PUVA treatment through your GP – this treatment is thought to be helpful for vitiligo sufferers.
- Concealers can help you camouflage the white patches. Contact the Cosmetic Camouflage Service, 28 Worple Road, London SW19 4EE, for advice on what products will work well, and what products are available on prescription. See also Chapter 13.
- Recent research carried out in Italy indicates that the anti-oxidant vitamins, A, C and E, together with the mineral selenium are helpful. You can buy a supplement called Selenium-ACE in Boots. See Chapter 8 for more details on anti-oxidants.
- For more information about vitiligo, contact the Vitiligo Society at 19 Fitzroy Square, London W1P 5HQ. Tel: 0171 388 8905.

SKIN CANCER

Skin cancer is increasing, not just because people are ignoring the warnings against sun bathing, but equally because more UV light is reaching us through the thinning ozone layer. And as we have seen, we British, with our characteristic types 1 and 2 skins, are particularly susceptible to the risks of sun-related skin cancer. Cases have grown rapidly in this country (it is the second commonest form of cancer in the UK), and there are now more than 40,000 new cases a year. However, it is reassuring to know that almost 90% of those who come forward for medical help have benign growths which are easily treatable.

We can fall victim to three different strains of skin cancer, all associated with exposure to sunshine. The vast majority of 'suspect' marks and moles on the skin represent the two less worrying strains (which, I hasten to add, are not types of malignant melanoma): basal cell carcinoma and squamous cell carcinoma. The most serious is malignant melanoma, and it is responsible for the majority of deaths from skin cancer.

So how can you distinguish between the three strains? Very broadly, the first two produce raised bumps which are more or less the same colour as the skin, and are found in areas that are normally exposed to sunlight.

Melanoma is quite different, and you will find a separate 'What to look for' list on page 71.

BASAL CELL CARCINOMA

This is also known as rodent ulcer and is characterised by raised little bumps which have a pearly look to them. They are commonly found on the face, particularly near the inner corner of the eyes and around the nose – you rarely find them below the neck. The bumps grow slowly for around six months and as they get larger, small blood vessels become apparent on the surface. In time these will break down into a crusted ulcer which does not heal of its own accord.

Treatment: A hospital will either arrange surgery or X-ray treatment – both are completely effective methods of curing basal cell cancer. Even more effective (with a 98% cure rate) is treatment via the Mohs Technique. Named after an American surgeon, this technique allows skin cancers to be removed accurately under local anaesthetic without the necessity of destroying healthy tissue to create a safety margin. The cancerous tissue is sliced off horizontally, a thin sliver at a time. The patient then waits while each sliver is analysed on the spot – and if more needs to be removed, it can be done so immediately. This technique is very effective for areas like the face, eyelids, nose, lips and ears, where saving healthy tissue helps avoid disfigurement. You can find out more about the Mohs Technique by sending off for a leaflet to the Imperial Cancer Research Fund, PO Box 123, Lincoln's Inn Fields, London WC2A 3PX. Tel: 0171 242 0200.

SQUAMOUS CELL CARCINOMA

Not as common as basal cell cancer, this strain usually develops on the neck, head and the back of the hands. It is also the type most associated with excessive exposure to sunlight.

Common early warning signals include the appearance of small rough slightly raised areas on the skin surface, known as actinic keratoses. These can disappear over a period of time if the skin is now protected from sun exposure, but if it continues to be exposed, they may develop into squamous cell cancers. These look like raised solid lumps which grow quickly and can double in size over six months.

Treatment: Mohs Technique (see above) or laser surgery to cut away the bump.

MALIGNANT MELANOMA

The name alone indicates that this is different from the other two types of cancer. A melanoma is a tumour which

70

arises from cells that produce melanin, the pigment that colours the skin and that is concentrated in moles and freckles. Unlike the other two forms of skin cancer, which are linked to long-term exposure of the sun, melanomas can be triggered by brief but intense exposure – particularly if it results in bad sunburn. A tendency to melanoma can run in families. Fortunately, it is comparatively rare.

Most melanomas develop on a mole, either a new one or an existing one, or a freckle. (Moles are raised, freckles are flat.) However, unlike a normal mole or freckle which always stays the same, a melanoma changes – in shape, colour or size. Women usually get them on the lower leg, men are more likely to develop them on their backs, but they can turn up almost anywhere – even on the sole of the foot.

If you have a large number of moles (over 100 if you are young, over 50 if you are older), or have several that are unusual in size, shape or colour, it is only sensible to keep an eye on them and watch for any change. If you are concerned about a mole, *don't delay in seeing your GP*. Early treatment is important, because some melanomas can develop very rapidly, and left unchecked the cancer can spread from the skin through the body.

Remember that malignant melanoma is rare and chances are that a biopsy will prove the mole to be benign anyway.

What to look for
• Changes in colour or shape
• Growth in size (especially any mole that grows to over seven millimetres – or roughly the size of the blunt end of a pencil)
• Itching, oozing or bleeding
• Any sign of inflammation or redness around the edge
• A mole that starts to itch or hurt

Treatment: The affected area will be cut away and sent for analysis to check whether it is malignant. Depending on how deeply the melanoma has penetrated the dermis, a skin graft may be needed. Follow-up treatment is essential to prevent recurrence of the melanoma.

SUN EXPOSURE FOR THOSE WITH SPECIFIC SKIN COMPLAINTS

Certain skin complaints can benefit from *carefully controlled* exposure to the sun – for others, like **cold sores** and **rosacea**, the sun can make the condition worse. As an example, sunlight can help dry up spots for some **acne** sufferers – though for a quarter of them, it can make the acne much more spot-prone. Some people find that their **eczema** is improved by the sun; again, others will find it makes their condition flare up.

Really, there are no hard and fast rules, but if you are one of those lucky enough to have your skin problems helped by exposure to the sun, make sure you go about it sensibly. The same rules apply as to people with skin types 1 and 2: limit your time in the sun, protect your skin and make sure you never get sunburnt.

Sunscreens can normally be used safely by everyone, but they do contain chemicals which can occasionally irritate **eczema**. If this is the case for you, try using a sunscreen containing titanium dioxide only, which reflects the sun off your skin and rarely irritates eczema. Likewise, there are some sunscreens available on prescription for people prone to sun rashes – ask your GP for advice.

Most **psoriasis** sufferers find that their condition improves a great deal when they are exposed to natural sunlight – if, for example, they have been on holiday. Many psoriatics find a spell on the Dead Sea (if they can afford it) can really help their skin. Below sea level, the damaging, burning UVB rays get filtered out of the atmosphere, which also explains why people can stay out for longer at resorts on the Dead Sea. Obviously, the same sunbathing precautions apply in the Dead Sea as elsewhere and extreme exposure is ill-advised. And for psoriatics, the soothing minerals and salts in the sea itself can sometimes bring remission of their problems for up to a year – but more of the Dead Sea in Chapter 13.

Light therapy: PUVA

Therapeutic artificial sunlight can help those with **eczema**, **vitiligo**, and severe **psoriasis** in a relatively short amount of time.

Known as PUVA, this is an effective and commonly used treatment which can only be carried out by a specialist, such as a dermatologist. It involves taking a psoralen tablet orally, and then, two hours later, receiving ultraviolet treatment to the body in a cabinet fitted with tubes that emit wavelengths in the UVA range – hence PUVA: psoralen plus UVA. The combination of the two treatments causes a substance to be produced in the skin which greatly slows down cell turnover. In all cases, the dose of UVA is very carefully recorded and kept within safe limits, and most patients are followed up long-term to assess any remote risks of skin cancer.

Sunlamps and sunbeds

Though similar, PUVA should not be confused with sunlamps and sunbeds. If you must use a sunbed, don't exceed a course of ten thirty-minute exposures *annually* and always wear goggles. Many dermatologists are concerned about the detrimental effects on those who sunbathe and then top up tans repeatedly with sunlamps and sunbeds – my advice would be to avoid them all together. You can achieve a tremendously good fake tan with one of the easy to use creams on the market if you want that golden glow. Remember, though, they offer no SPF protection, so you'll need to add that too if you go out in the sun.

PART 2

Self help and prevention

CHAPTER 7

Nutrition

We have seen in our discussion of individual skin problems just how important a balanced diet is to the skin's health. As the saying goes, 'You are what you eat,' – and that applies to drinking lots of water too! So which foods, if any, should you avoid – and which might actually help to heal your skin?

Basically, a good all-round diet which mixes proteins, fats and complex carbohydrates with essential nutrients, vitamins and minerals is what you need to aim for – not only for your skin's sake, but for your general health as well.

Research in the US has also indicated that out of a group of carefully monitored individuals, those who came forward with specific skin problems had a significantly higher intake of refined carbohydrates in their diet. By refined, we mean the sugary, starchy processed foods like cakes, buns, sweets and white bread (yes, all those seemingly delicious naughty foods), as opposed to the healthy complex carbohydrates which you find in foods like wholemeal bread, brown rice and porridge. Similarly, the volunteers were found to have a low intake of vitamin C. This vitamin, as we shall see in our next chapter, is vital for strengthening delicate blood vessels in the skin and promoting the healing of wounds. The researchers bumped up the group's intake of vitamin C, and after a year, the volunteers with skin problems were found to have a marked decrease in their problems.

TO DIET OR NOT TO DIET

You might find it worthwhile to do a checklist of your eating habits over a week or two, to see if there are any nutritional 'deficits'. Provided you are dedicated about detail, and interested in trying this, it might be worth employing the guidance of a dietician, to make sure you are doing it properly. Your GP should be able to recommend someone to you. If, by correcting the weak spots in your diet, you find that your skin starts to improve over a period of time – all well and good.

A word of warning, however. It is totally understandable to look to dieting if, having tried every lotion and potion on the market, you find your skin problem still rages. It is also true that food can occasionally cause an allergic skin reaction – as with **hives**, which we will discuss next. But just how important diet is in, say, treating **eczema**, **acne** or **psoriasis** is open to debate. Without doubt, a poorly controlled diet can aggravate chronic skin conditions, and even certain key foods like milk and eggs are often thought to exacerbate **eczema** for example, but bear in mind, cutting these foods out of your diet could lead to a nutritional imbalance – not to mention the time-consuming complications of checking the lists of ingredients on all processed foods. Again, I would advise you to follow a dairy-free diet only under the supervision of a dietician and only after having given topical treatments a fair trial.

Practitioners of TCM believe that **eczema** is caused by an internal 'overheating' and consequently they recommend reducing sugars, fats and alcohol while you are receiving treatment. In fact, drinking lots of water, for example when you drink alcohol, should balance things out – with the added advantage of staving off that hangover!

FOOD SENSITIVITIES

A number of skin disorders, however, are known to have a link to food sensitivities. Luckily, the trigger foods involved tend not to be nutritionally vital – their nutritional benefit can be culled just as easily from other foods, so eliminating them from your diet won't leave you feeling deprived or undernourished!

Hives
Those of you who suffer from hives (or urticaria) may find that eating strawberries, shellfish, eggs and nuts can trigger an attack. Perhaps monosodium glutamate – the flavour enhancer used particularly in Chinese food – is the culprit, and certain herbs and spices, like paprika, oregano, thyme and dill, may have an adverse reaction. Food colourants and flavourings, such as tartrazine and salicylates found in foodstuffs like ice cream and soft drinks, may have to be eliminated from your diet. The best way to be sure, is to keep a food diary, and eliminate one of these supposed culprits at a time. After a period of about a fortnight, reintroduce them into your diet, and if they set off an attack, you can be pretty sure you've found your enemy!

Cold sores
Chocolate, gelatin, seeds and nuts (especially peanuts, brazil nuts, almonds and cashews) are thought to be the culprit

foods for some sufferers of cold sores. One lady sufferer was brave enough to cut out all dairy products and milk especially, on the advice of a dietician. The cold sores disappeared and she is now back eating a small amount of dairy food with no ill effects. But if she eats a bar of milk chocolate followed by custard, she gets a cold sore the very next day. Opting for a dairy-free diet might sound rather drastic, and isn't necessarily the only answer for curing cold sores. Generally, as we explained back in Chapter 2, those who get plagued by cold sores tend to be run down anyway, and may therefore have neglected their diet. The same applies to **abscesses** and **impetigo**, both of which often indicate a poor diet. Herpes sufferers should also reduce stimulants like alcohol, caffeine, salt, sugar – and nicotine.

Rosacea

Certain types of food and drink may set off or increase the flushing of rosacea in some people. The following have been found to cause flushing and should be considered as possible trigger factors if you are having difficulty in pinpointing a cause:

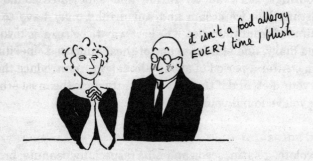

- liver
- steak
- spicy foods
- pickled, marinated or smoked foods
- yogurt
- sour cream
- all cheese (except cottage)
- chocolate
- vanilla
- soya sauce
- yeast extract
- dark vinegar
- aubergines
- avocados
- spinach
- citrus fruits
- red plums
- raisins
- figs

Before you flinch and gasp in horror (poor old chocolate looks like winning a prize for its evil effect on the skin!), bear in mind that any one of these foods has had an adverse effect on some people – but not all of them will be bad for you. If your rosacea is really troubling you, you could work your way through this list and eliminate each in turn. Depending on your life-style, you may find that it's the yogurt and cheeses and citrus fruits that you would miss the most – but there again, I might be completely maligning all you vinda-loo fans out there!

Alcoholic drinks, particularly red wines, tend to aggravate flushing, likewise caffeine.

FOODS FOR A HEALTHY SKIN

According to your individual preferences, try and get a good balance in your diet of the following:

- oily fish
- plenty of raw vegetables in the form of salads, crudités
- jacket potatoes
- brown rice
- porridge
- pulses and wholegrains – e.g. aduki beans, kidney beans, lentils, chick peas, tofu (all an excellent source of protein)
- most fruits, except perhaps citrus fruits if they are found to affect your skin
- lean meat like chicken
- lamb (lean cuts once a week)
- beef (once every ten to fourteen days)
- wholemeal bread and pasta
- avocado
- plenty of water, herb teas, vegetable juices
- dressing using garlic and olive oil

Actually, this dietary list would suit any individual, since it incorporates a lot of natural raw foods that will work their way through your system, helping to keep your bowels healthy as well as your skin. If you suffer from constipation on top of everything else, you may have noticed how this can make your complexion look extremely dull, so give those raw veggies a go! In their raw state, vegetables and fruit, sprouted grains and herbs are rich in nutrients and natural enzymes which are all sensational as skin fixers.

Avocados, for instance, are rich in vitamins A, C and E, some B vitamins, and potassium. And they're not to be missed if you are on a diet: half an avocado, with a drizzle of olive oil and a splash of cider vinegar, creates a good filling snack at only 200 calories. If you think even that is too much, mash the avocado with a spoonful of bio-yogurt and slap it on your face. Leave it on for fifteen minutes, rinse with tepid water, and you've just given yourself a soothing face pack – ideal if you suffer from itchy **dry skin complaints**!

You'll see I've listed **oily fish** as being good for you. Mackerel, salmon, sardines, herring, fresh tuna, trout and whitebait are all particularly rich in essential fatty acids which, as their name suggests, are essential to the many vital functions of the body (the heart in particular), as well as being important in maintaining a healthy skin. Essential fatty acids protect the lipidic barrier between each layer of skin, help to reduce water loss, and thus are important if you suffer from **dry skin conditions**. They also help to maintain collagen and elastin in the skin, both of which keep the skin looking youthfully plump and firm, and they play an important role in the circulatory system, as well as feeding the nerve endings and sensory receptors in the skin. However, if you really don't like oily fish in any form, try taking a **fish oil capsule** as a supplement.

Evening Primrose Oil is another excellent source of these 'good' fats – indeed recent studies have shown that both these supplements can be of benefit to **psoriasis** and **eczema** sufferers; nutritionists suggest that by decreasing our intake of animal fats and increasing our intake of fish and vegetable oils, we could achieve a marked improvement in eczemous cases, allergic conditions and inflammatory disorders. But more of EPO later.

Avoid
• All refined carbohydrates: found in cakes, white flour products, puddings, sweets, pastries.
• Excessive animal fats: cut down on whole milk (semi-skimmed is easy to adapt to), high fat cheeses, all fat on meat (game is better because of its lower fat content), butter and margarine, cream and ice cream. Stick to low fat yogurts if they don't upset your skin problem.
• Avoid too many canned foods.
• Avoid fried foods.
• Avoid sugary soft drinks, too much alcohol (the odd glass of white wine is fine), too much coffee and most chocolate unless it has a high cocoa content and therefore less sugar.
• Steer clear of barbecued, seared, burnt and highly spiced foods.

Doesn't sound too painful, does it? The most difficult part of going healthy will be getting rid of the refined carbohydrates – these quick energy snacks are often very tempting and tasty, as well as being ready to hand when you are suddenly hit with hunger. Try getting into the habit of carrying around a piece of fruit with you, or even a handful of raisins and some dried apricots, for those moments when your energy is low.

SPRING CLEANING YOUR INSIDES

Raw food days
Rather than opt for a long-term elimination diet, you might like to consider incorporating a 'raw food day' into your k. A marvellous way to cleanse the insides, detoxify the and keep the bowels healthy, thus in turn benefiting

the skin, eating purely raw foods is easier than you think. I'm not suggesting you tuck into raw liver, or go oriental and hit the sushi bar; on raw food days, you should aim to eat only fruits, vegetables and salads in their uncooked states. Obviously avoid citrus fruits if these are a trigger food for your skin condition, but otherwise feel free to eat as much as you want. Make sure you drink at least eight glasses of water as well.

Fasting

Once a month, you could try fasting for a day. This is when only liquids are consumed – no, not beer or tequila, but good old water, and preferably still spring water. Drink at the very least one and a half litres of the stuff – you can dilute with fruit juice to make it interesting – and don't exert yourself too much, since fasting can make you feel a bit feeble for a while. A quiet Sunday would be a good day to choose, rather than a busy day in your working week.

Juicing

Some people swear by juicing – a current fashion for sipping freshly squeezed vegetable and fruit juices which you stick to for a day or two as a detox diet. Obviously, to save your arm muscles, you would need to invest in a special juicer – although some softer fruits can be broken down and whizzed to a delicious pulp in an ordinary blender. Juicing to promote health and vitality has already taken the US and Australia by storm – and it now catching on in the UK as well. Certainly, the anti-oxidant vitamins (A, C and E) that are found in fresh fruit and vegetables can do wonders for boosting the immune system, combating illness and ensuring a healthy skin – but you shouldn't really overdo juicing. Although any excess vitamins and minerals will be excreted if not utilised, excess vitamin A (as derived from beta carotene in carrots) can accumulate in the liver over time, and will lead to dizziness, headaches and nausea. The answer is moderation – perhaps include juices in your normal diet, and make sure you vary your juices. Beginners should start with three glasses a day (8fl oz to a glass), drunk as soon as the juice is made.

CHAPTER 8

Vitamins and Minerals

Certain vitamins and minerals have been found to be helpful for problem skin conditions, but if you find the thought of a lot of pill popping too off-putting, look at the dietary suggestions instead. Again, a well balanced diet is what you should aim for – and foods rich in specific vitamins are listed at the end of each section.

VITAMINS

Vitamin A

Vitamin A acts as a barrier to infection as well as helping to maintain healthy skin. Many experts believe that this is a really important vitamin for those suffering from **eczema**, **acne** and **psoriasis**. In fact a deficiency in this vitamin results in hardening of the skin, similar to the skin of eczema sufferers.

It is also a powerful anti-oxidant. You may have heard talk about these anti-oxidants, of the importance of supplementing your diet with a combination of the 'supermodels' from the vitamin world – vitamins A, C and E, in order to stave off everything including, it seems, old age. In reality, anti-oxidants are very effective neutralisers of 'free radicals' – destructive and highly reactive molecules that are thought to be at the root cause of many very serious diseases like cancer and heart complications. Vitamin E, another anti-oxidant, is even thought to delay ageing *as well as* improving your sexual performance, but there is no evidence for this – and before you go mad stocking up on the stuff, do bear in mind that with all vitamins, you need to play safe and stick to the stated dose!

Beta carotene, derived from yellow vegetable sources (carrots in particular), is sometimes referred to as provitamin A. Basically, it consists of two vitamin A molecules joined together. This nutrient can help protect the skin from sun damage, and actually is an extremely safe way of supplementing your diet with vitamin A. The human body can readily convert beta carotene into vitamin A, and it is now known that people with high levels of beta carotene in their diets also have less chance of developing certain types of cancers than those with a lower intake of the nutrient. In contrast, an excess of vitamin A can lead to liver damage and scaly skin, and the vitamin should be avoided if you are pregnant or intending to become pregnant. An excess of beta carotene has no serious side-effects, though the skin might turn a slightly orange colour! Recommended daily intake: around 60mg.

Foods rich in vitamin A
Liver, egg yolk, margarine, butter, cheese, full milk, kidney, herring, mackerel; and beta carotene in spinach, sweet potatoes, carrots, pumpkin, mangoes, apricots, melons. (Lost by cooking any of the above at high temperatures and in fats.)

Vitamin C
It was the absence of vitamin C from the grim fodder of eighteenth-century seafarers that gave rise to scurvy: a

disease where there is haemorrhaging under the skin, where the gums bleed and the teeth fall out. After a medical experiment proved scurvy was a deficiency of vitamin C, English sailors took to carrying limes on board to supplement their diet – these 'limeys', as they were nicknamed, hoped to stave off future attacks of scurvy. And the craze has caught on – today vitamin C is the most widely used supplement of them all, even if we no longer fear a scurvy outbreak!

The vitamin is vital for skin health, in that it is important in the formation of collagen – the body's intercellular 'cement'. It also helps to heal wounds, repair tissues, and stimulate the production of white blood cells. Equally, vitamin C is a powerful anti-oxidant.

It is quite a fragile vitamin and vulnerable to light, heat and air, so you must store your pills in a cool dark place. It also can't be stored in the body, so you need to ensure a regular intake: around 50mg a day should be enough (although some researchers would like to see the figure rise to 100mg). Alternatively, eat five portions of the following fruit and vegetables a day, and you will be getting around 100mg anyway.

Foods rich in vitamin C
Most citrus fruits (choose from another food if you can't tolerate citrus fruits), brussels sprouts, potatoes, tomatoes, green leafy vegetables, green peppers. (Use foodstuffs when fresh and don't overcook. Store in a cool dark place.)

Vitamin E
For post-operative wound healing, prolonging cell life, protecting against neurological disorders, improving skin condition and poor blood circulation, this powerful anti-oxidant is

recommended. As good for the skin is vitamin E in ointment or cream format – remarkable for its softening and healing properties. All kinds of skin problems, from the **very dry** to the **very oily**, can be helped by topical application of the vitamin. Equally, you will find plenty of skin creams containing vitamin E on sale in health shops.

As a supplement, you could take vitamin E in a multivitamin formula, since large doses are unnecessary and could give rise to unpleasant symptoms. Levels over 300mg a day have occasionally been associated with symptoms like fatigue, nausea, palpitations, and a mild blood pressure increase.

Foods rich in vitamin E
Cold-pressed oils (e.g. vegetable oils), nuts (especially almonds), egg yolks, brown rice, asparagus, wheatgerm.

The B complex group of vitamins
Thiamin (B1)
Riboflavin (B2)
Niacin (B3)
Pantothenic Acid (B5)

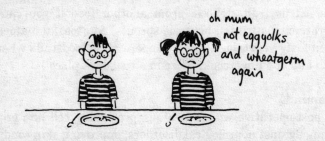

Pyridoxine (B6)
Folic Acid (B9)
Cobalamin (B12)
Biotin (also known as vitamin H)

Each of the B vitamins has a slightly different role to play in maintaining a healthy system, but they also work together to promote, among other things, healthy skin. Taking one capsule a day providing 25–50mg of each vitamin should be fine if your skin is generally in poor condition; and you should maintain this supplement for three months. People with skin problems often have a deficiency of these B vitamins; they are vital for skin repair, and preventing rashes, cracks, itching and scaling, as well as sores. Generally, B vitamins are entirely safe – even in quite high doses, though very high doses of niacin (about 3.6g per day) may cause liver damage – and the supplement is best avoided by people suffering from the following: gout, stomach ulcers, liver disease, diabetes.

Foods rich in the B group of vitamins
Besides the natural sources, many breakfast cereals come fortified with niacin, riboflavin, B6 and B12 – and you might find thiamin and niacin in certain white and brown flours – wholemeal flour automatically contains these two vitamins. Otherwise, eat plenty of dark green vegetables, seeds, nuts, wholegrains, meat, eggs and potatoes.

MINERALS

Zinc
Symptoms of zinc deficiency span **acne**, **dry** and excessively **oily skin**, to slow healing of wounds and persistent

infections. Also, without zinc, vitamin A cannot be properly utilised, so make sure you are getting plenty of this mineral. Rather than take a supplement, your best bet is to introduce lots of fresh foodstuffs into your diet, since zinc is negligible in highly refined foods.

Foods rich in zinc
Meat, poultry, fish, seafood, milk, yogurt, cottage cheese, beans, pulses, wholegrain foods.

Calcium
A vital mineral, calcium works with vitamin C in the manufacture of collagen. It is necessary not only for strong teeth and bones, but in maintaining a healthy skin. Without it, our nerves would fail, our skin and muscles would lack tone, wounds wouldn't heal and blood vessels would be weakened.

Foods rich in calcium
Milk is an obvious source, but if you are allergic to cow's milk, there are plenty of other sources of calcium which you should include in your diet. These include: cheese, nuts, canned and fresh fish, root vegetables, green vegetables, oatmeal, eggs.

Selenium
We need only tiny quantities of this mineral, but it is important for maintaining healthy skin and hair, and for staving off **dry** flaking **skin conditions**. It also plays an important anti-inflammatory role in the body and works with the anti-oxidant vitamins C and E in helping to protect the body from major diseases. As long as your diet is rich in the following, you probably won't need to add a selenium supplement.

Foods rich in selenium
Kidneys, brazil nuts, oily fish, bread, rice (particularly brown rice), eggs, shellfish, fruits and vegetables.

KEEP IT SIMPLE

If you suspect yourself of having a serious vitamin or mineral deficiency, you should see your GP. In other cases, rather than single out each vitamin and mineral, and thus run the risk of confusion, huge expense and possible overdosing, try to take a compound supplement which contains a number of the minerals and vitamins we've already discussed. Above all, make sure your diet is rich in those foods which are vitamin packed!

CHAPTER 9

Traditional Chinese Medicine

Sally's story

'I suffered from shingles a few years ago – actually, the attack was pretty bad, with a nasty rash that covered quite a lot of my body. I had been to my GP for help, and he had prescribed a topical steroid cream which did in fact get rid of the rash – but I was left with more pain than I'd experienced with the rash. I went back to my GP, who told me I had post-herpetic neuralgia. Rather depressingly, he said there wasn't much he could do about it, bar giving me painkillers. He said I would have to learn to live with it. My tongue had a weird greyish-black coating which worried me, but by this stage, I was prepared to seek alternative help.

'I had a consultation with a traditional Chinese practitioner, who asked me loads of questions. He wanted to know what my skin rash had looked like, and I told him it had been red and blistered, with an intense burning pain accompanying it. The doctor told me that I was suffering from "damp heat" – essentially, that's the heat produced by the amount of pain I was experiencing, plus the damp coming from the water in the blisters. The cream my GP had prescribed may have cured my rash, but it had increased the pain, and that was trapped more deeply into me because the "fire" was drying the damp, and creating more heat. My blackish tongue he explained as "the ashes formed by heat rising from a fire". It all sounded terribly gobbledegook and, funnily enough, terribly logical too – anyway, suffice to say, I was willing to let him treat me.

'Through the position of the shingles, the doctor was able to pinpoint the source of the "fire" as being in the liver and the gall bladder. Had my shingles been elsewhere, the medicine he prescribed me would have been adjusted accordingly. The doctor prescribed herbs that would help to expel the damp through the urine, the bowels and through the skin – eventually cooling the body down. A few sessions of acupuncture accompanied this, to open up the "meridians" and so help expel the heat.

'Feeling very ignorant, I asked what the meridians were. The doctor explained that you enter the body's energy network via **acupuncture** points – there are about 800 in the body. These points join to form twelve major channels or "meridians" that run symmetrically through our bodies and which are named after the organs to which they are attached. When these are manipulated, you can influence the energy and balance in the system.

'Over a period of time, my tongue slowly turned from yellow, to white, and finally to a normally healthy pink colour. The pain disappeared, and I haven't had a recurring attack of shingles either – I think it's a miracle really.'

Traditional Chinese Medicine (or TCM) can do wonders for skin complaints like **eczema**, **psoriasis**, **dermatitis**, **acne**, **rosacea** and, as Sally's story tells us, **shingles** too. In fact, Chinese herbal medicine has been curing these conditions for over 3,000 years – so, as they say, there must be something in it!

What is Traditional Chinese Medicine?

In Traditional Chinese Medicine, a holistic approach is used – which means that it treats the whole body, not just part of it. Actually, the philosophy behind TCM is quite interesting. We humans are viewed as a microcosm and indeed a reflection of nature. All of creation is made up of a marriage of opposites – Yin and Yang – cold and hot, dry and wet, body and mind, inner and outer. Harmony in this union of opposites equals good health. Chinese medicine even uses aspects from the natural world as labels for upsets that occur in the human body. For example: heat is manifested in the skin when it gets red and hot to the touch. 'Wind' is found in movement in the bodily changes: for example when skin eruptions change location and itching strikes. Dampness, as Sally found out, relates to oozing skin eruptions, swelling, pus and blisters – the body is not performing healthily in moving fluids properly around the system, and so they accumulate in the skin.

As Sally describes, **Chinese herbs** are an integral part of TCM – they include the use of roots, flowers, leaves, bark and minerals. The herbs are used both internally and externally – internally they are cooked up by the patient in boiling water for half an hour or more, and drunk as a tea, or sometimes taken in tablet form. Externally, the herbs are used in creams, lotions, compresses and washings, all specially prepared by the pharmacist according to ancient Chinese prescriptions. These will help to relieve the itching, cracking, redness and blisters that accompany your complaint.

A patient's internal organs (lungs, liver, gall bladder as well as blood) would be assessed, because it is believed that all these organs influence the condition of the skin. TCM believes that most skin conditions reflect an imbalance

within the body itself – and this imbalance is the *cause* of
the condition. The *symptoms* of the imbalance are what
you can see: the rash, the scales, the flaky skin and so
forth.

Any disorders raging away on the inside of the body, as in
Sally's case, may also be tackled through **acupuncture** – so
that the life force or energy known as 'chi' which flows along
the meridians can be strengthened and freed from any
blockages. Any obstacle to this vital energy flow can lead to
disharmony and eventually disease, so redressing the flow
from the start of treatment will help the body to support
itself for the future.

At the same time, **herbal medicine** helps to alleviate
the external *symptoms*. Follow-up treatment, be it a
course of massage or meditation, concentrates on improving your **life-style**, through getting regular relaxation,
never eating anything very hot or very cold, and alleviating stress, which is often seen as having a detrimental
effect on skin problems.

What happens at a TCM consultation?
Visiting a traditional Chinese physician is completely
different from visiting your GP. You probably won't have
to give a urine or blood sample, you won't see a stetho-
scope – and you will probably be asked a load of questions
that might not seem entirely relevant to your skin problem. You should go with a fairly empty stomach, and any
alcohol, food or drinks that colour the tongue should be
avoided. Make sure, too, that you inform your doctor if you
are seeing a practitioner of Chinese herbal medicine,
especially if you are currently receiving treatment from
your GP.

Many factors such as past illnesses, your age, your

emotional well-being – even the number of children you have, will be taken into account. From the moment when you first enter the room, the doctor will be taking note of how you hold yourself, what your posture is like, the state of your complexion and the brightness of your eyes – truly a holistic approach!

Your **tongue** is another important tool in diagnosis. Practitioners in TCM regard the tongue as extremely important, since it is the only organ on the inside of the body that can be viewed with ease from the outside. The tongue is connected to each meridian in the body, and so to every organ in the body. Its size, colour, moisture content, shape and the quality of the coating are all taken into account as indicative of the health or otherwise of the internal organs.

Your **pulse** is important too. Six pulses are taken: three on each wrist using three fingers. On the left wrist, the first finger detects patterns from the small intestine and heart. The second finger, from the liver and gall bladder, and the third, from the kidney and bladder. On the right wrist, the physician can detect the state of your lungs, your large intestine, the spleen and the stomach. What he or she is looking for is an abnormal rhythm. The pulse may be choppy or deep, wiry or slow.

And of course, as well as this, your **skin condition** is carefully examined, so that the physician can prescribe a combination of tailor-made herbs for you to take over a period of time. Depending on your condition, this can range from a few weeks, to a few months.

Why use acupuncture for skin complaints?
When acupuncture is performed, some chemical substances in the spinal cord and brain are released into the body – and

among these substances is the tongue-twisting adrenocorti-cotrophic hormone – one of the components which take part in the formation of a steroid. From orthodox medicine, it is known that steroids can have a beneficial effect on many skin diseases, so when this natural steroid hormone is released and activated through acupuncture, the body is stimulated to heal itself.

What exactly is acupuncture?

Acupuncture is an integral part of TCM and helps to re-establish the correct flow of energy along the body's meridian channels: essentially, it helps get your insides sorted out so that your outside can be healed in the long term. Fine stainless steel needles are used – these are carefully inserted into your skin at the vital 'acupuncture' points. Each point has a particular function which, when stimulated and in combination with other points, can act a bit like a combination lock on a safe: twiddle the right set, the door blows open – and hey presto – you can get to work on the treasure! In acupuncture, the points work together to restore the balance in your energy pattern.

On average, between three and six treatments will be necessary before a noticeable improvement takes place, but if the thought of needles is off-putting, rest assured that you're not about to undertake a form of torture more suited to a horror movie – amazingly, acupuncture doesn't really hurt at all. Most patients experience the sensation of a slight pinprick – a tingling sensation, that's all, and a feeling of pressure. When correctly done, there won't even be any blood, and the sensations disappear very quickly. The dispos-able needles used are very fine indeed, and are inserted into the skin at an oblique, vertical or almost horizontal angle. Usually, only a tiny part of the needle goes into the skin.

Variations on acupuncture include: acupressure (where fingers instead of needles are used on the points), stimulating the points using a mild electrical current, or using balls of dried herbs on top of the needle's handle which are then set alight. A gentle heat is produced which passes down the shaft of the needle and increases the effectiveness of the stimulation.

Melanie's story
Eight-year-old Melanie suffers from **atopic eczema** – it's a condition she's had since babyhood. Her mother Angela has long since learnt what things affect eczema: from wind, soap powder, bedding and food, to dust mites, cold weather and sand in the summer. On top of this, Melanie occasionally gets an asthma attack. It is a hard life for a little one – and night-time brings no relief. Eczema itches, and on hot nights, that itching is aggravated by sweat and the myriads of unseen house mites.

A few months ago however, Melanie tried Traditional Chinese Medicine. The doctors prescribed an indescribably bitter mixture of herbs prepared into a soup – but after two doses a day for a week, Melanie was sleeping through the night and her itching was fast disappearing. This encouraged her to keep drinking the concoction, even though she found it so distasteful. Six weeks later, and her body no longer had open sores, and by late autumn, her skin was a healthy pink, and clear.

CHINESE HERBS FOR ATOPIC ECZEMA

Atopic eczema is an exceedingly common disease in children all over the world – and in temperate climates like the UK, figures are particularly high. TCM is having dramatic effects in improving the condition, as Melanie's experience shows – and similar success stories have been monitored over the last ten or so years by Dr David Atherton, consultant dermatologist at Great Ormond Street Hospital and a specialist in childhood eczema. The effectiveness of TCM was first revealed to him when a child with severe atopic eczema under his care was taken by his parents to see a Chinese doctor – Dr Ding-Hui Luo, in London's Chinatown. The child was treated with a daily 'tea' prepared from dried medicinal herbs, and the treatment was immediately and impressively effective with no obvious side-effects. From that point on, Dr Atherton suggested to parents of children with atopic eczema which was proving unresponsive to conventional therapy, that they might also consider taking their child to Dr Luo. The parents reported back to Dr Atherton, and in a group of thirty children, substantial improvement was observed in around 80% of the cases.

Inspired, Dr Atherton set about concocting a fixed prescription of Chinese herbs in the form of a mini pill made up of dried herbal concoctions, to replace the traditional tailor-made prescription. The purpose was to produce something that was more palatable than the bitter teas of old, and equally could easily be handled by pharmacists – also, that could be readily prescribed around the country. Currently, the formula is available in granule and powder format, under the names Zemaphyte or Phytopharm Eczema Granules, but as yet the formula does not have a licence. Your dermatologist will advise you whether or not the granules would suit your condition. Alternatively, the National Eczema Society has an information sheet entitled 'Chinese Medicinal Plants for Atopic

Eczema' which gives up-to-date advice on the treatment for eczema sufferers.

Above all, the traditional scepticism of Western doctors towards anything 'alternative' is breaking down, if a little slowly – and that has to be welcomed. Collaboration between Eastern and Western approaches, as exemplified by Dr Atherton's research, is on the increase and again is something we should welcome, given the extraordinary success stories of TCM.

How much does treatment cost?

Chinese practitioners' fees vary – but a typical first consultation may cost around £40 or more; after that, fees tend to drop to around £20–£25. A week's supply of herbs can cost from around £20–£40.

That sounds expensive – can I get TCM on the National Health?

It is rare – but some hospitals are offering both acupuncture and Chinese herbal medicine in their clinics – your GP can

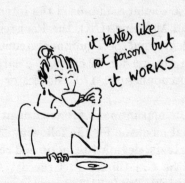

it tastes like rat poison but it WORKS

advise you here. If you suffer from **severe eczema** and are referred to a dermatologist, they may recommend you try Zemaphyte (see above), but even then, it can work out at about £375 for a month's supply, as it is not yet available on the NHS.

If your GP refers you to an acupuncturist and you have private medical insurance, you may be able to claim costs.

How do I find a good practitioner?

Before you make an appointment with a practitioner, make sure they have recognised certificates of qualification. At present there is no legislation to stop anyone setting up a practice, and since herbs can be dangerous if wrongly prescribed, you need to be very careful about who you see.

Even though herbal remedies are natural, they can cause dangerous side-effects in some people – such as liver damage. Your best bet is to see your GP first before undertaking TCM. The National Eczema Society has an information leaflet on Chinese medicinal plants for **atopic eczema**, and they too can advise you about suitability.

You can get a copy of the Register of British Acupuncturists, which also combines details of the International Register of Oriental Medicine (UK), the Register of Traditional Chinese Medicine, and the Traditional Acupuncture Society, by sending a cheque for £2.50 plus a large SAE to the Council for Acupuncture, 179 Gloucester Place, London NW1 6DX.

To make an appointment for treatment by traditional Chinese herbal medicine for the following skin complaints: **eczema**, **psoriasis**, **dermatitis**, **acne** and **rosacea**, you can also contact the Chi Clinic, 10 Greycoat Place, Victoria, London SW1P 1SB. Tel: 0171 222 1888.

CHAPTER 10

The Helping Herb

When we think of herbs, we think of those lovely aromatic plants which can help transform plain food into mouthwatering concoctions. But many familiar herbs also have the power to heal our bodies. Using herbs in healing is as old as time, and today, more than half the world's population relies on them for health. In our previous chapter, we saw how TCM uses complex herbal remedies to help treat skin disorders successfully – and though it may surprise you, herbs also form the basis of most Western modern medicines, with currently more than 100 prescription drugs based purely on plant and herbal extracts.

TCM, as we saw, is an extremely effective if complex and sometimes foul-tasting route to problem-free skin, but there are some simpler remedies that you could concoct yourself. Bear in mind that herbs are very potent, and have to be respected and used correctly for successful results. Like anything else, they can be harmful if used incorrectly or taken in excess. (Some herbal preparations should be avoided if you are pregnant.) Herbs can be taken in many different ways using varying parts of the plant. You can take them internally as an infusion, tablet or capsule, or externally as a poultice, essential oil or tincture.

Remember that herbal remedies will only be truly effective if

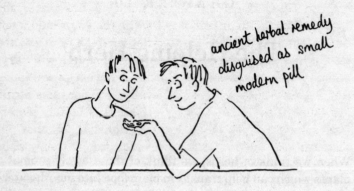

ancient herbal remedy disguised as small modern pill

your diet is balanced and healthy – a condition that is essential anyway for skin health. If you are in any doubt about your food, check back to our chapter on nutrition.

Dosage
If you are treating children with herbal remedies, the dosage should be halved, or for toddlers, kept to a quarter of the adult's dose. Ideally, of course, you should consult a medical herbalist who will be more skilled at ascertaining accurate dosages, and you should always tell your doctor if you are taking herbal preparations as some can interact badly with conventional medicines.

PREPARATIONS

Internal: as a 'tea'
Herbs taken internally are either in the form of infusions or decoctions.

With an **infusion**, the water-soluble parts of the plant are extracted by steeping the plant in hot water for approximately fifteen minutes – rather as you would a pot of tea. The leaves of the plant, whether fresh or dried, are best suited to this process. Quantities of course will vary, and to be safe, you should consult a herbal practitioner (see Useful Addresses), but generally, infusions use about 1oz (30g) of the herb, to 1 pint (600ml) of boiling water. Use a covered container for the infusion, so that no essential oils are lost through evaporation – then strain and drink when warm.

Decoction remedies consist of a liquid made by simmering the herb in water – the ratio is usually one part plant to twenty parts of water. This is the method best suited for bark, roots and seeds which should be crushed first into small bits, and left to soak for ten minutes or so. Simmer the pieces for around fifteen minutes, and leave to steep for a further ten minutes before draining, and drinking.

External: poultices
Particularly good for easing pain and inflammation, old-fashioned poultices comprise a wet softish heated mass of herbs which you apply directly to the skin. The usual preparatory method is to crush fresh herbs with a little moisture – enough to make a paste – and this is placed between two pieces of muslin. The warm paste 'bag' is then held onto the skin for about ten minutes.

Both: Tinctures
Tinctures are basically concentrated solutions of the appropriate herbs, which have been steeped in alcohol. The latter acts as a preservative, and tinctures are usually taken in tiny doses. It is probably easiest to buy the tincture of the

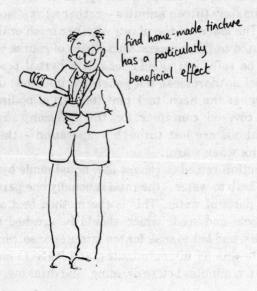

I find home-made tincture has a particularly beneficial effect

herb you want, and a good health food shop will have a list of stockists for you, or try contacting a good herbal suppliers directly, such as G Baldwin & Co, 171–173 Walworth Road, London SE17 1RW. But if you prefer to make your own, place 4oz (100g) of the herb (usually leaves) in a sealable bottle with ¾pt of either gin, brandy, rum or vinegar. Leave for a fortnight, making sure to shake the bottle each day – then filter the contents through a fine cloth and store in a dark glass bottle.

Capsules, tablets and **essential oils** really are best left to the experts, unless you've plenty of time on your hands and a penchant for fiddly processes!

HERBAL CHECKLIST FOR SPECIFIC DISORDERS

herb	complaint	method/product
Aloe vera	burns, chapped and dry skin, dermatitis, eczema, sunburn	creams, lotions, gels
Borage	eczema, psoriasis	Aru Herbal Products have creams, oils, shampoos, etc, available from Holland & Barrett
Burdock	dry and scaly skin conditions such as psoriasis and eczema	use root and leaves, and as a poultice for boils (excessive daily use is thought to be bad for liver – use occasionally)
Dandelion	warts and blemishes	use the root of plant
Echinacea	sores, eczema, sunburn, herpes simplex	externally as a poultice or tincture
Fenugreek	inflamed and infected skin	use seeds as poultice
Hawthorn	psoriasis	as a 'tea'
Horehound	skin irritations, bites	as an antiseptic used externally
Lavender	burns, scar tissue	apply oil neat
St John's wort	psoriasis, external wounds	as an oil or poultice

herb	complaint	method/product
Sarsaparilla	psoriasis, eczema	use liquid extract topically
Slippery elm	boils and abscesses	powdered bark used in a poultice
Tea tree	athlete's foot, boils	as an oil applied in diluted form externally
Witch hazel	inflamed skin, sores	as an astringent
Yarrow	dry, irritated skin	infuse leaves in olive oil and apply externally

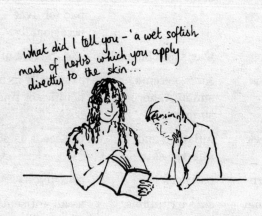

what did I tell you – 'a wet softish mass of herbs which you apply directly to the skin...

CHAPTER 11

Homeopathy

Lesley's story

'My husband Tom and I taught English in Cairo when we were first married. It was quite a stressful time for me if I'm honest. I didn't enjoy teaching much, the men were a nuisance because of my blonde hair, the noise and the dirt used to get me down. Anyway, when we came back to the UK, I started to develop clusters of raised pimples which were incredibly itchy and almost looked like a heat rash. They gradually spread all over my body – except, amazingly, my face. I had never had anything quite like this before, except as a teenager, when I had a rash on the side of my mouth which lasted for years. It was a bit like a cold sore, in that it would crack open and weep, although I had it diagnosed, and they told me it wasn't a cold sore. I was given steroid cream, which in retrospect I feel just suppressed something which was to come out at a later date. The only other significant factor from my past was my brother, who had asthma.

'Anyway, back to this rash. It went on for a year. I couldn't wear short-sleeved clothes, the spots itched like mad and they wept. I went to my GP who didn't know what it was. He sent me to the Royal London Skin Hospital where I had to wait for ages, in a corridor full of people itching away like

111

me! Eventually, I was seen by a lady Chinese doctor who told me I was incurable. She said the problem was in my blood and I would have it for life. She thought it was some kind of eczema. She gave me two enormous pots of lanolin cream and told me never to use soap in the bath again. I remember smearing this greasy stuff onto my body and sitting in a bath full of tepid water and bursting into tears, thinking this was it for the rest of my life.

'After that, Tom's family suggested I try homeopathy – something they were all very keen on. I went back to my GP for a referral to the Royal London Homeopathic Hospital – I didn't just want to pick any old practitioner, and at that hospital, they've trained as conventional doctors before studying homeopathy, so they really know their stuff. I had

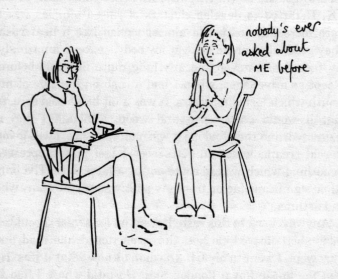

nobody's ever asked about ME before

a wait of about two to three months, but the end result was fantastic. I saw this very nice sensitive doctor, and he looked at my body and talked to me for about two hours. He asked so many questions, odd things like, "Does beautiful music make you cry?" and "When you see a crooked picture on the wall, do you want to straighten it?" I suppose he was getting a whole picture of me. He prescribed Pulsatilla in pill form, and within two weeks the rash had started to go, and by six weeks it had gone completely. All that was left was a wart on each thumb. I went back to him and said that his treatment had been brilliant, but look! He prescribed something else, and they eventually went as well.

'I now use homeopathy all the time, and for my children too. Interestingly, a couple of weeks after my son Oliver was born, he developed a total body rash. We were away from home at the time, and a local GP prescribed a steroid cream which I really didn't want to use. When we got back home, I took him off to the Royal London Homeopathic Hospital and they said that he had obviously got it from me and he was working it through his system. They gave him the same treatment and it disappeared.'

What is homeopathy?
Homeopathy, which has been around since the time of the ancient Greeks, is basically the medical practice of treating like with like. By that, we mean treating an illness with a substance which, if taken in large quantities by a healthy person, would produce symptoms similar to those of the illness it is used to treat. When minute quantities of that substance are taken by the sick person, it miraculously helps the body to throw off the illness – a sort of natural healing process, in effect.

There are now five homeopathic hospitals in Britain – and

113

some GPs also practise homeopathy. Look in any local chemist and it won't be unusual to find a stock of homeopathic remedies on the shelves – Boots, as an example, even have their own brand of remedies. All this is great news if, like Lesley, you have got nowhere with conventional medicine. The other huge plus about homeopathy is that the remedies can treat both psychological and physical symptoms simultaneously, and given the role stress plays in exacerbating skin problems – not to mention the deep-seated fear and self-loathing you may be burdened by on top of your skin condition – this has to be welcome news.

As Lesley found, a consultation with a homeopathic practitioner can be a very relaxing and fulfilling experience. You really feel that here is someone who has got time for you, who regards your worries and low self-esteem to be of equal importance as the state of your spots. Or, to put it another way, your own weeping is as significant as your weeping sores! Given the pressure our dermatologists are under to whisk patients through in double quick time, the homeopathic approach is infinitely preferable. Like conventional medicine, you will need some follow-up appointments – some practitioners like to see you every four to six months, even when your condition has cleared. Incidentally, it is not a good idea to undertake homeopathic treatment if you are currently receiving **acupuncture** or using **steroid creams** since these may interfere with the flow of energy – and it is also best to reduce your intake of caffeine.

Like TCM, homeopathy views skin disorders as the outer manifestation of some inner imbalance in the body. Some skin conditions lend themselves to self-prescription, and we list them opposite. However for chronic skin conditions, and initially anyway, it is advisable to see an experienced homeopathic practitioner.

HOMEOPATHIC SELF HELP FOR SPECIFIC SKIN PROBLEMS

The following are often used for the listed specific skin conditions, and are readily available from chemists. Remember to follow the instructions on the bottle with regards to dosage.

Boils and abscesses:	Belladonna, Hepar sulph., Mercurius, Silica, Lachesis, Arsenicum.
Impetigo:	Graphites, Rhus tox., Mercurius, Antimonium crudum.
Warts:	Dulcamara, Antimonium crudum, Nitric acid, Causticum.
Shingles:	Iris versicolor, Lachesis, Rhus tox., Arsenicum.
Ringworm and athlete's foot:	Arsenicum, Graphites, Sepia.
Hives:	Urtica urens, Apis.

For **eczema**, **psoriasis** and **acne** you should always consult an experienced practitioner.

For a register of doctors, contact The Royal London Homeopathic Hospital, Great Ormond Street, London WC1N 3HR, or The British Homeopathic Association, 27a Devonshire Street, London W1N 1RJ. (Send SAE.)

CHAPTER 12

You, Your Skin and Your Relationships
And How to Cope with Stressful Situations

Sally's story

'When I was a teenager, I was incredibly shy. I have a beautiful older sister which didn't help my confidence much. Liza was, in my eyes, brilliant, kind, beautiful and constantly in demand as far as boys were concerned. I, on the other hand, was spotty, dull, plump and fifteen. I got **acne** at the age of fourteen, and despite periods when it seemed to clear up, it lasted right through my teens. It got worse before parties, typically – and I didn't help matters by picking at my spots, which left my skin looking sore and raw. I felt no boy would ever want to date me.

Actually, that turned out to be untrue. When I was sixteen, I met a boy called John on a weekend music course. He played the violin, and I played the clarinet. We had a lot of interest in common – *and* he had spots too! Though we never talked about our spots, it was like some tacit understanding. We saw each other after the course, but it didn't last that long. I remember some boys sniggering behind our backs at a party. They shouted out, "Look at those two! Talk about zit features!" It cut right through me. I became very introspective, and hardly went out through my college years. I just assumed everyone would find me unsightly. I can honestly say that my skin condition scarred me for life – and I'm not just talking about the physical symptoms.'

Sad, isn't it? Sally's story is sad, and all too common. Whether it's **acne**, **eczema**, **psoriasis**, or even the lone pimple and wayward wart – suffering from a skin condition can make you feel like a real outsider.

Why do skin sufferers feel bad?
Well, the answer lies partly in the fact that ever since the biblical leper, the medieval plague and the Victorian pox, we have been handed a series of vivid impressions and prejudices to cling on to as far as abnormal skin conditions go. And even today, in our so-called enlightened times, most people equate an abnormal skin condition with something nastily infectious, so chances are you are going to get stared at a great deal. Worse still, people might avoid you all together. Understandably, this is going to make you feel hurt, angry, rejected – full of vengeance probably, even if you only want to express that vengeance by sticking your tongue out!

It is entirely natural for you to feel upset by other people's ignorance – and hurtful comments, like being called 'poxy, spotty or scabby' especially during those sensitive teenage years, can be very painful stuff. It doesn't help your confidence and feelings of 'acceptability' either, that though people can't 'catch' your **psoriasis** and **eczema**, you may find yourself being asked to leave a swimming pool, or not to take a shower in your local gym. It is tough, but given that treatment for your skin condition can be long term, you will have to learn how best to cope with other people's insensitive reactions, and how to build up your self-esteem.

Ashley Medicks, the founder of the newly formed charity

Skinship and himself a sufferer of the relatively rare mycosis fungoides, believes that public reactions of disgust have 'conspired' to disable people with skin disease. He describes his own feelings of isolation – comments which I am sure will ring true to anyone with a significantly visible skin condition.

'You [the public] tend to catch sight of us and then you look away. Your expression asks the question when you stare: "What is that?" "Is it infectious?" "How can you live with that? – yuk! You poor thing!" The emotional turmoil is also enormous. It is bad enough having to cope with the physical consequences – but what makes it so much worse, is when agoraphobia, discrimination at work, family dissolution and divorce result directly from being a skin sufferer.

'The thing about skin problems is that they tend to look worse in the bath, because the skin gets red and angry. You feel filled with self-disgust, and like some modern day leper. I was looking at my own skin in the bath, and it was shouting at me in its redness and ugliness, and it did so in such a vehement way that I couldn't ignore it. I felt despair for what seemed like the first time and I cried. The tears turned to anger and frustration, and I began to think that if it was this bad for me, with all the support I have from my wife and friends, what must it be like for those suffering alone.'

Let's do exactly that – let's hear it from one who suffers alone. Sarah suffered from **eczema** very badly as a little girl, and now her four-year-old son Jason is a sufferer. Her husband has left her, and she feels very guilty about Jason's condition and frustrated that there is no one to offer support.

Sarah's story
'The name calling was the worst thing when I was a little girl. You feel nobody loves you. You feel ashamed and dirty.

I was called everything from "scabby" to "flaky" – and now I feel so bad that poor Jason might have to go through all this, and in some way it is my fault.

'The sheer daily routine of looking after a child with a skin problem is a nightmare – especially when there is no supportive partner to help. Every day, I have to vacuum the house, for fear of dust or house mites – every night, Jason's hands and feet have to be bandaged up to try and stop him scratching. The poor little chap nearly goes mad with wanting to scratch – sometimes he gets away with it, and attacks his skin till it bleeds. The creaming and bandaging can take up to two hours at a time. I feel tremendous anger sometimes, and occasionally I want to yell at Jason to stop scratching – but you can't do that.

'I hate people staring at Jason – and then staring at me – and you know they're thinking that I've hit him or even poured boiling water onto him.'

HOW TO COPE WITH THE OUTSIDE WORLD

Understanding 'the enemy'
Other people's insensitivity is a tough nut to crack. And yes, it might seem an odd thing to do, but if you can try and understand why some people act as if without thinking or feeling, the chances are their comments and rebuffs won't hurt quite so much. If you think about it, it is only human nature for people to stare at the unfamiliar. Think about road accidents – and how, intellectually, we know it is unnecessary and insensitive to look, and though we don't like ourselves for doing so, the urge to look is powerful.

The public look upon skin diseases with fear. Perhaps they

recall childhood memories of illnesses that were accompanied by a rash, and how frightening that had seemed at the time. Try remembering that when people seem aggressive or evasive towards you; generally they are acting out of fear. Now that's not to say you are a frightening spectacle, but that they are frightened because they don't know how to react to you. Skin abnormalities strike a deep fear in many people – and this fear could also hark back to the time when lack of hygiene did indeed give rise to poor health and diseased skin, when the affected person would be cast out from the community, as lepers once were. There is even a name for this defensive attitude to skin disease: it's called the leper complex.

On the occasions when you catch sight of revulsion in someone else's eyes – well, that's a different matter altogether. It is upsetting, hurtful and angry making. But if you do ever get the chance to talk about your skin problem to one of these 'leper-phobes', you will be amazed how much it helps. And yes, I admit, taking the initiative in first meetings may seem an intolerable responsibility. 'They should accept me as I am' is a common excuse, but not a very understanding one. If you can learn to offer reassurance, that will be much more productive. Make sure you talk to the 'enemy' for the right reasons – not from anger, but from the point of view of informing. You might, for example, like to point out to them that many spots and rashes are neither infectious nor contagious – and **acne** is at least proof that your sex hormones are very much alive, if kicking a little too actively!

Ideally, what you need is recognition, by those who appear to rebuff you, that fear and repulsion are totally inappropriate responses. This comes down to putting you in the role of a teacher, which you perhaps hadn't banked on! The need to educate the general public into better awareness of skin abnormalities, and the deep need sufferers have for psychological support and understanding is tremendous. And it is not just the general public who need educating, but doctors, nurses and health administrators too. When someone with a skin problem goes to their GP or medical centre, it isn't always helpful to fob them off with a prescription for antibiotics – a more 'holistic' approach, discussion of stress levels and contact with fellow sufferers are all important too.

The power of the group

It is a sad fact that some sufferers have avoided relationships because of their skin condition, and some have even been driven to suicide through a sense of acute isolation and despair. But having a skin problem needn't mean you have to be an outsider – far from it. As with any minority group (though with near-on 8 million sufferers of skin conditions in the UK alone, minority sounds almost something of a misnomer!) the power of identification that arises when fellow sufferers get together can be tremendously therapeutic. Sharing problems, letting all those years of hiding and anger come safely out into the open, offering support – even laughing in the face of adversity can be healing stuff indeed. The newly established charity Skinship, as an example, is aiming to establish a nationwide network of local support groups for sufferers. At these groups, or 'dos' as they will be called, the aim is to develop feelings of solidarity, warmth and support, as well as helping sufferers with problems like body image and lack of confidence. You can write to Skinship to find out if there is a group in your area – or even if you fancy starting one yourself.

The address is Skinship UK, 10 Thurstable Way, Tollesbury, Nr Maldon, Essex CM9 8SQ. Tel: 01621 868666.

Acne, eczema and psoriasis sufferers already have their own supportive societies which you can contact. They each provide stacks of information on the individual condition as well as organising social contacts and local group support. The addresses are as follows:

Acne Support Group, PO Box 230, Hayes, Middx UB4 9HW. Tel: 0181 845 8776.

National Eczema Society, 163 Eversholt Street, London NW1 1BU. Tel: 0171 388 4097.

The Psoriasis Association, 7 Milton Street, Northampton NN2 7JG. Tel: 01604 711129.

YOUR SKIN, RELATIONSHIPS AND SEX

In a recent survey conducted by the University of Wales at Cardiff, 84% of **psoriasis** sufferers said the worst aspect of their condition was the difficulty it caused with relationships. Three out of five people with **chronic eczema** felt their sex lives had suffered because of their skin problem, according to a survey conducted by the National Eczema Society – and over half said that eczema had affected their choice of career, with just under half saying they had lost some income in the last year as a direct result of their condition – the average loss being a staggering £7,200 a year.

The evidence is plain to see. Constant itching and embarrassing skin soreness can play havoc with your career and your relationships. Small wonder that it takes an awful lot of courage to go out and meet people! Couple that with what in your mind is a completely disfiguring skin condition, and the courage needed to socialise takes on epic proportions.

In a way, we are all conditioned into believing that in

order to initiate a relationship, you need to be in possession of a few, albeit ridiculously unattainable, 'starter points'. For example, it is taken as read that skin and hair play quite an important role in sexual attraction and self-confidence – so even the solitary common cold sore can be seen to be detrimental to the dating game (remember Sarah's story?) especially given its prominent position around the mouth and on the lip!

However, having a skin condition doesn't mean that it is impossible to have close long-lasting relationships as well as lots of friends – and if that is what you want, you might find the initial support of a 'skin group' to be of great help. Within that friendly and supportive environment, you can learn to make friends, trust, grow confident, swap tips, and indeed socialise. Don't forget that a really worthwhile relationship goes much deeper than looks alone, and once people get to know you, they will not even notice your skin.

All this might sound easy and trite – but if you don't give people a chance, you won't achieve anything. It is particularly tempting for teenagers plagued with acne to lock themselves away, assuming that unless they look like extras from *Baywatch*, with slim, perfectly proportioned figures and blemish-free filmstar looks, no one of the opposite sex is going to give them a second glance. In fact, to dispel one myth, there are plenty of actors and stars, from Michelle in *EastEnders* to *Yes Minister*'s Paul Eddington, who cope with very visible skin conditions, proving that 'acceptability' has nothing to do with how pimple-free you are!

If you do get rejected by someone you are interested in, try not to jump to conclusions by assuming it is because of your skin. People say no for all sorts of reasons. However, if someone refuses you because of your skin condition, explain to them that it has nothing to do with dirt, nor is it infectious. If they still don't want to know – they're simply not worth bothering about, however alluring they initially might have appeared!

Obviously, if you have a skin condition that affects a large part of your body – and particularly the visible bits (face, hands, neck), you are going to have a tougher time of coping socially than if your condition appears only in small patches. Having said that, some sufferers who may just have a little patch of **eczema** behind the knee can be totally devastated by this. Basically, how well you cope comes down to body image and self-esteem. Once you are trapped in fear, in believing you are going to repel people, there may seem no way out.

The work of Changing Faces

If all this sounds familiar to your story, you may like to get in touch with a support system like that offered by the charity Changing Faces. The primary focus of this organisation is to offer practical advice, help and training in 'social interaction skills' to anyone affected by disfigurement, especially facially. Clients, be they burns sufferers, those with birthmarks or other visible skin conditions like **acne** or **eczema**, are given careful assessment, individual counselling, and help in a whole range of relevant skills. Workshops with fellow sufferers will help you build your confidence and break out of your fear about meeting people. There are more specialised workshops where you can learn assertiveness skills, stress management and relaxation, how to build better relationships, as well as touching on questions of intimacy. For young children, coping with facial disfigurement poses an immense challenge, and there are separate workshops where your child or teenager can learn how to deal with everything from shyness and bullying, to coping with teasing and how to boost self-esteem.

You can contact Changing Faces at 27 Cowper Street, London EC2A 4AP. Tel: 0171 251 4232.

Rebuilding self-esteem

Sometimes it is hard to give yourself credit for being the interesting, witty, intelligent, kind and fun person you are – if your skin leaves you feeling 'written off' in the looks department.

Seeing your skin problem as a challenge rather than a disaster can have tremendously positive results – but it takes courage to highlight your other attributes in social situations, rather than relying on your looks as many people do. Taking the initiative really can pay off. Remember that other people may feel embarrassed as to how to talk to you – you can defuse that, by approaching them first. Listen to Paul's story about how he felt on first talking to Anne – an **eczema** sufferer in her twenties:

'I just didn't know how to talk to her when we were introduced at a party. Was it polite to address her hair rather than her face? That seemed condescending – was it better to be aggressive and stare boldly? After a while, the conversation seemed to flow pretty easily, and I can honestly say that I stopped seeing her skin, and started to see her. We had loads in common – and I was grateful that she was so forward and easy to talk to; normally I hate talking to people at parties! Anyway – six months down the line, and we're an item!'

Try remembering that your problem, by being highly conspicuous and out in the open for all to see, can work to your advantage. Unlike psychological and emotional problems which are equally numerous but effectively hidden from the world, you have the golden opportunity to widen other people's understanding of skin conditions. Less conspicuous problems, in contrast, may never surface or get explained – as a result they may fester, leaving the sufferer feeling bitter and isolated. In a way, particularly with regard to social gatherings of any kind, your skin condition is encouraging you to 'act' extrovertly, and this can only be to your advantage. By displaying your essential personality and worth through your actions, you don't have to depend on your looks and your face – and people will like and admire you for it.

Sex
Within a sexual relationship, certain skin disorders can cause problems. **Psoriasis** and **eczema** as an example can leave you feeling itchy, sore, irritable and plain worn out – hardly the ingredients needed to induce either tender or passionate lovemaking! **Eczema** can make you feel as if you cannot bear to be touched, and often the itching is worse at night-time; **acne** and **cold sores** can make you very self-conscious about kissing. In these circumstances, you have to be honest with your partner in as gentle a way as you can, without it sounding like a rejection of that person. Try explaining to your partner how you feel. Suggest that perhaps a cuddle is all you want – often a cuddle can be even more intimate than full intercourse. Explain to your partner what makes you itchy and what feels fine. Perhaps he or she can help you apply your soothing creams.

Some people find that a shower or bath after sex helps remove any irritation and itching. Again, you have to be sensitive about this. Leaping out of bed and heading straight for the shower might be misinterpreted, so perhaps you should explain beforehand how washing can help your condition. And if you feel itchy or sore in the genital area, consider using a lubricant like KY jelly. Alternatively, if symptoms persist, you should see your doctor. This is particularly important if you have **genital warts**, which are caused by a different kind of virus from the common wart or verruca (see Chapter 2).

CHAPTER 13

Skin Therapy

HOW TO MAKE BATHING EASIER

Let's be honest: one of the worst aspects of chronic skin conditions like **eczema** is having to take a bath. No, not because you don't want to get clean – but all the complications of soap-free bathing, hard water, soreness and sticky creams tend to turn what should be a relaxing ritual into a nightmare. Even for those of you out there with less chronic conditions, bath-time can quickly turn into blues time, especially if you hate having to look at your body in the nude.

But bath-time needn't be a chore. It is really a question of finding the right bathing agent to suit your skin condition. If you have **irritant contact dermatitis** or plain **dry skin**, you should avoid soap as it has a very drying effect on the skin. Likewise, especially for those of you with **contact dermatitis**, you may react badly to fragranced soaps. Some soaps are advertised as having anti-bacterial ingredients suitable for **acne** sufferers, but since the soap is in contact with the skin for such a short time, they can't really have a long-lasting effect – far better to use an anti-bacterial preparation after cleansing.

Using bubble bath or bath salts (as I found to my cost) is

not the answer either – they can really leave your skin feeling scaly and scratchy. Bathing in water alone is also very drying and no way to get clean – even if you may have passed an enjoyable twenty minutes with your plastic duck. So what's the answer?

Substituting soap with bath oils and creams which are added to running water will help your skin to retain moisture. Some will even coat the body in a film of oil which helps to seal in water and thus reduce irritation. To prevent the oil from being removed, you should pat the skin dry with a towel, rather than opt for a vigorous rub-a-dub!

As long as you pick a hypo-allergenic product (Boots stock plenty of suitable oils and creams: Wash E45, Bath E45 and Unguentum Merck are excellent), your **dermatitis** should prove less troublesome, and you may find you can swap over from potent steroid-containing preparations as a result. Wash E45 and Bath E45, as an example, are both non-drying alternatives to soap and can be used on the face and the whole body. They can be used for all skin conditions, including **eczema** and **psoriasis**. Of course you can get certain medicinal bath oils on prescription, but for the sake of your morale, I would ask your GP for non-lanolin-based ones which you have to apply before getting in the bath (remember Lesley's story?). Some are awfully difficult to remove from the skin's surface, and besides, a lot of people find applying sticky gunge to a dry body extremely distasteful.

Bath water generally should be lukewarm rather than either hot or cold; this is because an extreme change of temperature when you get out of the bath can set off itching. If your skin is raw and sore, if you suffer from **eczema** or **psoriasis**, bathing can be really painful to start with. Cut down on the amount of time you spend in the bath, or shower using a gentle spray as an alternative to bathing. **Psoriatics** and those with **dermatitis of the scalp** often find that shampooing with a preparation containing tar (Polytar or Capasal) will improve their condition. Tar has antiseptic and healing properties, and can help soften thickened skin and remove scales. It is important to leave the shampoo on your hair for a period of time – your doctor will tell you exactly how long and how often to use it. A simple ointment like white soft paraffin will also remove excess scaling after a bath. Anti-fungal shampoos can greatly improve **seborrhoeic eczema**, and these are readily available. Neutrogena's T/Gel is also a good therapeutic shampoo to choose and is suitable for **psoriatics** too.

Acne
Because of the myth that acne is a dirty skin condition, many poor teenagers spend their time overwashing, which actually makes matters worse. It can lead to the skin becoming too dry and certainly sore. Also, it is better not to use facial scrubs or strong astringents if you are also using a preparation containing benzoyl peroxide, since they can cause irritation. A gentle washing and cleansing routine is what you should aim for, to help remove excess oil. There are some good medicated washes on sale; really you need to experiment to find the right one to suit you.

Impetigo and cold sores
As these conditions occur mostly on the face, it is best to use a dermatological washing cream like Wash E45, followed by Zovirax or whatever preparation has been prescribed by your GP. Most importantly, don't let anyone else touch your towels or flannels as both conditions are highly contagious.

Post-bathing moisturisers

There is a wide range of moisturisers and nourishing preparations aimed at women in particular – many of which also purport to do wonderful things for the skin, including miraculously reversing the ageing process and at the same time giving us the complexions of a supermodel. Would that they could! The more expensive the cream, the more the manufacturer seems driven to blind us with scientific jargon. Indeed, it was only a few years back that the wording on some expensive creams had to be changed to conform with new laws akin to those demanded by America's Food and Drug Administration. Instead of stating that a cream 'reduces' wrinkles, manufacturers must now say that a cream reduces 'the appearance of' wrinkles: effectively, it's all in the eye of the beholder! Only something which invades and alters the deepest layers of the skin, the dermis, can really have any effect on wrinkles – as with surgery, for example – so these creams were initially guilty of false promises.

The hype still continues, though. You may have seen creams or facial treatments which list **collagen** as a major ingredient. The claim is that the collagen will penetrate the skin and plump and firm up wrinkles. Collagen can only work at plumping up wrinkles when injected into the skin (as we shall see in our next chapter), since its structure is such that deep penetration is impossible when applied superficially; as one nurse qualified to administer collagen explained to me, these claims are like saying you'll be able to push a tennis ball through a fine mesh!

Unfortunately, however, British women's skins tend to age faster than many others – faster than Japanese, American, French or Italian skins – and sadly, manufacturers know that women are vulnerable when it comes to those first signs of ageing, and they seem only too willing to exploit our vulnerability. We will look at some affordable and not so affordable tricks you can employ if you really are keen to hold back the years, but ageing is essentially the pull of gravity at work. If you want to avoid wrinkles entirely, you need to live in space!

So do you need a moisturiser at all? And does expense equal extra efficacy? Moisturisers are actually valuable for all skin types – and all skin problems. With our centrally heated environments and polluted atmospheres, moisture is constantly being drawn out of the skin – hence the need to put moisture back. Basically a good light moisturiser like those made by Neutrogena or Vaseline should be used after bathing, but avoid lanolin-based ones if you have **dermatitis**, since it can make the condition worse.

Even though **acne** is an oily skin condition, you still need to keep the skin moisturised. Oil-free gel moisturisers are good because they add water and not oil, and tend to be soothing and calming on the skin. Heavier, thicker moisturisers should be avoided by those with **acne**-type conditions, since they can leave the skin greasy and clog the pores.

EVENING PRIMROSE OIL

It's been hailed as the wonder supplement – nature's cure-all for women. Maybe you are already familiar with the well-publicised powers of Evening Primrose Oil – perhaps it's already bringing you relief during those intolerable days running up to your period. I know that for me, the supplement helped tremendously with one symptom of PMS – namely painfully tender breasts; some women find it even helps their mood, alleviating those awful feelings of irritability and depression. Having said that, it annoys me that the price of such relief is so high; Evening Primrose Oil currently enjoys a market in the UK worth well over £30 million, easy money made from women's misery – that's how I see it!

So what is the Evening Primrose, what exactly are its health-giving properties, and how can it help your skin? The oil comes from a plant not unlike a common primrose, but one that only blooms between five and seven in the evening (hence its name). The Evening Primrose is a North American native and it thrives in extreme weather conditions. Though it is easy to mistake it as today's wonder drug, its powers can actually be traced back some 7,000 years to the days when Amerindian medicine men made poultices from its leaves to soothe sprains, and used the seed pods as an anti-inflammatory infusion. EPO's success today is dependant on those very seed pods. They contain an oil rich in an essential fatty acid called gamma-linolenic acid, the same fatty acid that is found in human breast milk – but let's call it by its easier initials, GLA.

EFAs and GLAs

Essential fatty acids (EFAs) are needed by the skin to help maintain its tone and elasticity. In fact, the first medical experiment on Evening Primrose Oil which took place in the 1960s revealed that when rats were fed a diet lacking in EFAs, they experienced hair loss and skin problems. Our chapter on nutrition has already stressed the importance of a diet rich in EFAs (plenty of oily fish, seeds and olive oils). To redress this, half the rats were fed linoleic acid (an EFA found in polyunsaturated vegetable oils), and the other half were fed GLA from the Evening Primrose plant. The results were hugely significant, especially for the treatment of all kinds of skin problems. The rats fed GLA recovered far quicker than the other group, and evidence showed that GLA was more effectively used by the body for repairing damage then EFAs.

Actually GLA is produced naturally by the body from linoleic acid found in foodstuffs like green leafy vegetables, oils, seeds and pulses – and given our penchant for heavily saturated fats, our diet is often deficient of GLA. Some foodstuffs like processed vegetable oils, which are a mix, even interfere with the enzyme that converts the linoleic acid in our bodies into GLA. Far better therefore to opt for safflower, rapeseed, sunflower, walnut or soyabean oil for your salads and cooking, all of which contain EFAs.

Interestingly, one British chemist discovered that certain widely differing conditions, ranging from **atopic eczema** to diabetes and PMS, all derive from the body being unable to convert linoleic acid into GLA. To correct this deficiency, a good source of GLA is needed – as found in Evening Primrose Oil and, incidentally, even more so in borage oil, though this oil is, as yet, not so readily available.

Evening Primrose Oil and the skin

Dry and ageing skin
The skin is very sensitive to nutritional deficiencies, and watching what you eat is fundamental to improving **dry skin conditions**, and in general to keeping the skin looking youthful and healthy. Indeed, many people complain about dry skin and scaly patches when they follow a low fat diet, so don't be tempted to forego your suppleness in favour of skinniness! The EFAs found in oily fish etc. help maintain

the water barrier between the skin's cells, and when skin becomes dry, it isn't oil that's lacking but water. Many dermatologists remain sceptical about the effect of EPO on your skin – but equally many partakers find that taking EPO daily helps keep skin moist – you can even pierce a capsule and smooth the oil directly onto your skin, or mix it with a little moisturising cream. I mix mine with a little Nivea. It's a far cheaper and in many ways more effective skin food than those expensive creams and potions!

Acne and oily skin
If you've got acne, you probably think that the last thing you need is an oil of any sort coming into contact with your skin. However, Evening Primrose Oil can help to redress the balance of sebum in your skin. Some brands also contain vitamin E which is a great skin healer, and lecithin which helps to clear waste matter from beneath the surface of the skin. A 500mg capsule a day should be taken.

Psoriasis
Trials conducted with psoriatics over a period of eight weeks showed moderate improvement in 60% of cases given EPO as a supplement. There is no evidence to show that EPO has a dramatic effect on psoriasis, but it is something you may like to try in addition to other recommended treatments.

Eczema
Essential fatty acids play an important role in cell health, and when people are fed a diet containing no EFAs, they quickly develop eczema-type symptoms. Likewise, it has been found that the enzyme which converts EFAs into GLAs

in the body is particularly inactive in eczema sufferers. Since this was revealed to the scientific and medical world, there have been hundreds of trials involving EPO and eczema sufferers; one of the most publicised reported a significant improvement in **atopic eczema** in sufferers taking 4,000mg a day over three weeks (2,000mg for children). Itching was reduced, as was scaling and redness – all by approximately 30%. This is terrific news for those with eczema, and if you fancy trying the same for yourself, don't be put off by the vast dosages required and the thought of huge bills at your local pharmacist: EPO is now available on prescription for those with eczema. Ask your GP for Epogam.

Again, EPO can also be applied externally to the most affected parts of your skin. Squeeze out the contents of two capsules for a soothing balm to help relieve the itching and scaling. It is also safe enough to use on babies and small children. Liz Earle, in her booklet 'Evening Primrose Oil', suggests making up your own eczema skin oil – again, safe for babies. She herself suffered from eczema and found that it cleared up through daily doses of EPO.

Eczema skin oil
1 tbsp calendula oil
1 tbsp St John's wort oil
1 tsp wheatgerm oil
1 tsp Evening Primrose Oil

Mix all the above ingredients together and store in an airtight jar away from direct light. This nourishing oil contains vitamin E, essential fatty acids, and soothing herbal compounds, and helps relieve itching and scaling.

For more information, contact the Evening Primrose Oil Office on 0181 743 1335.

TEA TREE OIL

You've probably heard a lot of talk about tea tree oil or you may have noticed it on sale in the Body Shop; like me, perhaps you were initially puzzled – doesn't tea grow on bushes rather than trees? Well, yes, and no. The tea tree in question, whose oil has become such a wow as a topical antiseptic, is native to the northeast coastal region of New South Wales – in fact, so special is this plant that you can't find it anywhere else in the world! The tree is actually pretty small and the leaves are the part that is used medicinally. The oil from the leaves has been used for centuries, crushed into a sort of tea by aborigines, and it was even added to beer by Captain Cook and his crew on the *Endeavour*.

In the 1930s there were some impressive medical reports of its benefits: tea tree oil was reported to dissolve pus, leaving infected wounds clean and bacteria-free. Nowadays, you don't have to collect and crush leaves from the source – tea tree oil comes ready for topical application and is ideal as a skin disinfectant for **acne**, **athlete's foot**, **boils** and **carbuncles**, **cold sores**, **impetigo**, **psoriasis** and **ringworm**, as well as burns and bites. The oil penetrates the skin easily and is non-irritating if not used excessively. Use the oil occasionally and simply follow the instructions on the bottle.

GOODBYE PROBLEM SKIN, ALOE VERA

Aloe vera – no, it's not the cry of Bet Lynch as she greets Vera Duckworth across *Coronation Street* – even if it comically sounds that way. Aloe vera, the cactus-like plant which also belongs to the lily/onion family, is already known for its moisturising properties. Now it has become widespread as a wonder treatment for anyone with problem skin. Aloe's healing properties have actually been in use for thousands of years. Taken internally, the juice can help with irritable bowel syndrome, sciatica, ME, hernias and arthritis; externally, in its gel format, it has had astonishing success with sufferers of **eczema**, **psoriasis**, **acne**, **hives**, **impetigo**, **dermatitis**, **boils**, **warts**, **abscesses**, bites, burns and cuts – indeed, every skin complaint you can imagine! Research in the Ukraine has revealed that aloe vera contains a hormone in its gel that can accelerate healing in wounds and third degree burns – and such is the faith in this extraordinary plant, that the American military stockpiled the gel for use on wounded soldiers during the Gulf War.

So what makes it so magical? The juice is rich in anti-oxidant vitamins and has nine out of the ten most important amino acids, plus a wide range of trace element minerals like calcium, chromium, copper, manganese, magnesium, zinc and potassium. On top of this, aloe vera contains saponins which have antiseptic properties, and anthraquinones, which have anti-viral, anti-inflammatory and antibiotic properties. It is reportedly helpful in rebuilding tissue through encouraging cell regeneration.

Aloe, taken as a tonic, and topically as a gel, is obviously worth trying if other preparations have had no effect on your skin complaint. It is non-toxic, but equally some general skin care products which claim to contain aloe may have only 2% of the plant in them, and any preparation needs to have at least a 30% content in order for it to take effect.

You can buy the pure juice from health food shops – the taste is rather pleasant, like a sharp lemon juice.

MAKE-UP AND CAMOUFLAGE FOR PROBLEM SKIN

When your skin problem spreads to your face as well as your body, it can really knock your confidence for six. People may tell you you're pretty or handsome, but it is probably the last thing you feel. If only some magic potion could hide that rash or those spots . . . Well, in a sense, make-up can do just that! Contrary to popular myth, make-up rarely causes spots – and it can in fact be an excellent way of disguising your skin condition and in turn boosting your self-confidence.

Obviously you need to be careful to pick make-up that will suit your skin type. Those that are specially formulated for oily skin, for example, will be less likely to clog the pores and aggravate **acne**. You might have noticed that some cosmetic products carry the label 'non-comedogenic' – this effectively means non-clogging, and if your skin is prone to oiliness then these products will be entirely suitable for you. Remember to remove any make-up thoroughly at night with a cleanser that leaves the skin feeling soft, not greasy.

You can also get skin-toned blemish sticks for disguising individual spots – these might be better than covering your whole face with a thickish foundation which can leave the skin looking sallow over a period of time. They are also very effective in that they often contain drying agents and antiseptics which will speed up the healing of individual spots.

Eczema sufferers can also wear make-up – but the number of products you can use is somewhat limited. If your skin is red and weeping, you shouldn't put any make-up on it at all until the rash fades. The best advice is: test make-up on small patches of skin before buying. Most good cosmetic counters will let you do this – some may even have samples that you can take home and try. Wait twenty-four hours and if your skin doesn't react adversely to the make-up, all well and good. Some people with **eczema** find they can't tolerate foundations as these can irritate the skin. Lipsticks, nail varnish and lanolin-based products, as well as perfumed cosmetics, may all sensitise the skin.

Used on particularly troublesome patches specially formulated camouflage cosmetics are helpful if you have **rosacea**, broken veins, **vitiligo** or persistent **eczema** on the face and hands. There are a number of different products available, in a wide variety of tones to suit your skin – and some contain sunscreens and are waterproof as well, so you can even swim in them.

Cosmetic camouflage service
The Red Cross offers a cosmetic camouflage service for people with severe skin conditions, scars, birthmarks and disfigurements, especially those that affect your life-style, but you need to be referred by your GP. The volunteers all have experience of working in the Therapeutic Beauty Care Services to which the Red Cross service is affiliated.

Consultations last about forty-five minutes, during which time your skin is colour matched with a cover cream. As the creams contain over 38% pigment, they are much denser than ordinary foundations. The make-up process of mixing and setting is shown step-by-step – and after that, you can go about your daily life without the fear of people staring at you.

For more details, contact the Cosmetic Camouflage Service, 28 Worple Road, London SW19 4EE. Tel: 0181 944 8909.

AROMATHERAPY

Can rubbing essential oils into your skin really help clear your skin disorder? Given that problem skin is often a visible reflection of an invisible or internal imbalance, aromatherapists believe that massage, baths and compresses with essential oils are an especially helpful solution, because they have a deep effect on both the physical and emotional well-being of the individual.

A professional aromatherapist will help you overcome the root cause of your skin condition – and he or she will probably prescribe creams and oil blends that you can continue to use at home. The therapist will want to know not only about your symptoms, but also about you as a person. You will be asked about your diet, your life-style, the stresses and strains on your life, and only once a vivid picture has been painted, will appropriate oils be prescribed. Because these oils are so powerful, you must always use a professional aromatherapist and ideally consult your GP beforehand, in case your particular skin condition is allergic to these highly fragranced products. You can find a professional aromatherapist in your area by sending an SAE to the Register of Qualified Aromatherapists, PO Box 6941, London N8 9HF.

What are essential oils?
Essential oils aren't oils in the greasy sense – they are highly concentrated, volatile substances which represent the most potent form of a plant's aromatic and fragrant materials. The oils come from the flowers, leaves, bark, wood and stems of the plants. Sometimes, you need huge amounts of the raw ingredients, just to produce a few drops of oil – hence the fact that they are expensive and considered precious. Some act as

a tonic, some as a sedative, and nearly all of them have
antiseptic and anti-viral properties. If you are buying your
own, only get the best and go to a reputable source. Keep the
oils in dark bottles, stored in a cool dry place, with the caps
tightly closed to avoid evaporation. They keep quite well for
three months.

Oils for specific skin conditions

complaint	*essential oils often used*
Acne/oily skin	juniper, bergamot, tea tree, lemon, sandalwood, camomile
Rashes/allergies	lavender, melissa, camomile
Dermatitis	lavender, camomile, patchouli, juniper, rosemary, benzoin
Burns, sores and cuts	lavender, camomile, geranium, tea tree
Psoriasis	tea tree, bergamot, benzoin, geranium, lavender
Eczema	lavender, camomile, juniper, patchouli, bergamot, geranium
Cracked and dry skin	carrot seed, neroli, frankincense, geranium, camomile, benzoin
Infectious skin conditions	lavender, bergamot, peppermint, sandalwood, tea tree, lemon, rosemary
Athlete's foot	myrrh, patchouli, tea tree, lavender
Stretch marks	neroli, mandarin, lavender

How to use the oils

Essential oils are rarely used neat. In massage, aromatherapists blend a few drops of each with a carrier like a vegetable oil – the best are virgin cold-pressed oils which contain active vitamins but do not have their own smell. The most commonly used carrier oils are walnut, wheatgerm, sweet almond, grapeseed, soya and hazelnut. Use the appropriate oils every day for around six weeks.

Massage: Useful for most skin conditions except open sores, infectious or inflamed problems. First blend three or four drops of each oil into two teaspoons of carrier oil, then bribe your husband, wife, partner or friend into giving you a soothing massage!

In the bath: After running the bath, add about six drops of oil and soak yourself for about fifteen minutes. Don't use soaps, cleansers or other oils – keep the windows closed, and relax.

As a compress: Useful for inflamed and infectious skin conditions. Add three to four drops of essential oil to a bowl of warm water. Soak a flannel in the mixture and place over the affected area. Cover with a towel and leave for at least two hours.

As a facial steam: To open pores and release impurities, fill a large bowl with hot boiled water and add ten drops of essential oil. Drape a towel over your head and hold your face over the bowl for five minutes.

FACIALS

And talking of facials, I expect like me, you've found yourself wandering around a large department store, only to be cornered by a white-coated cosmetics girl, offering you a free facial and consultation. Facials have become the buzz word of the beauty business – but do they actually do any good?

Essentially, modern skin care products can be soothing, comfortable and pleasant to use – and I feel the psychological benefit of having someone cleanse, moisturise and massage your skin, providing this doesn't kick start an irritation, has much to recommend it too. For those of you with **dry skin conditions** in particular, a facial every two or three months will do wonders for your particular problem. It is like giving your skin a super boost: dead skin cells are removed through deep cleansing and steaming, the skin is fed with moisturising packs – and an hour of doing nothing is tremendously helpful for those worry lines!

In addition, localised massage relaxes the facial muscles and improves circulation: in fact, it is something you could do for yourself – all it takes is three to five minutes every evening before you go to bed; look for a good massage instruction book in your local library, and simply use your favourite emollient.

Professional facials vary tremendously, though each beauty therapist or salon will tend to use just one make of skin care products. Professional facials are not cheap – ranging in price from £25–£40 for a forty-five-minute to ninety-minute treatment. However, there are two that I would highly recommend for their professional and medical awareness of the properties of individual skin types, together with their effectiveness in treating dehydrated skin: the Clarins and Mary Cohr range of facials. If you have a beauty salon near you, and some spare cash for a special treat, they are well worth splashing out on!

LIFE FROM THE DEAD SEA

In Chapter 4, we mentioned how therapeutic a visit to the Dead Sea is proving for sufferers of **psoriasis**. Some psoriatics can get remission from their problem for up to a year or more, following a few weeks by the Dead Sea. What makes the region so special for people with skin conditions is the unique combination of soothing mineral salts, together with the fact that its low position means the burning rays of the sun are filtered out of the atmosphere. Obviously, you should still wear sunscreens – but this kind of environment is ideal for psoriatics, and indeed all skin sufferers, since you can safely shed your clothes and so receive the positive, beneficial side-effects of ultraviolet light without fear of burning from excessive exposure.

The healing powers of the Dead Sea have been acknowledged and recorded since biblical times. In fact, our beauteous friend Cleopatra used to bathe here – and her skin was renowned for its perfection! The sea itself is really a vast inland 'lake', some 1,300 feet below sea level. Situated in the eastern part of Israel, it is the lowest place on the earth's surface, and also one of the hottest. Such an intense heat throughout the whole year causes massive evaporation to take place, and this enormous loss of water is replaced by the River Jordan and also by numerous springs that have a very high mineral content. The water is an almost totally saturated solution, in fact – which is why you see bathers floating on the surface without any effort whatsoever.

The mineral salts of the Dead Sea have high concentrations of magnesium, calcium and potassium chloride. In addition there is a higher concentration of bromine (psoriasis sufferers have a lower level of bromine in their bodies than others), which, with trace elements, helps to stimulate the natural repair processes of the body.

No one knows exactly how the salts do their magic, but psoriatics report a marked improvement in scaling skin, aching joints and most particularly, the distressing symptom of itching. Apart from these obvious advantages, keen Dead Sea goers benefit as much from the camaraderie of being in the company of fellow sufferers and the freedom, too, to walk around without clothes, and without the fear of being stared at. As Ashley Medicks recalls:

'People are embarrassed at first, but you soon lose that. The place has a unique sociable atmosphere and you can soon forget about yourself. Something special happens when skin sufferers get together – they only stare at you to ask interesting questions about your condition – not because they are disgusted by it.'

There are special 'skin' package tours to the Dead Sea – and you can find out more about these from the Psoriasis Association. VIP Holidays, as an example, have a special Health Holiday Department and boast over thirty years of experience with psoriasis sufferers. You can contact them on 0181 952 2059. Unfortunately, not everyone can afford three weeks plus by the Dead Sea. In contrast, our lucky European neighbours actually get to receive treatments in one of the many clinics dotted around the shores of the sea, courtesy of their own NHS – but no such luck here, of course!

However, there are DIY kits you can buy, like those from Finders International's range of Dead Sea mineral skin care products. You can buy Dead Sea mineral salts quite cheaply from health food shops, which are added to a bath of lukewarm water. When the minerals have dissolved, soak in the bath for twenty to thirty minutes, rinse with fresh water, towel dry and apply a mineral-rich moisturising agent. Wrap up, keep warm and relax for thirty minutes. Used three times a week over a four-week period, the salts can improve skin conditions tremendously.

Finders have a helpline you can call for free advice on skin problems, and how to use their products. The number is 0580 211055.

CHAPTER 14

The Beauty Business

Tempus fugit

You may remember back at the beginning of the book, some talk of a protein substance called collagen. Collagen is like the mortar in the bricks and mortar of our skin's composition. And it's that network of interwoven fibres of collagen which holds the dermis, and the epidermis on top of it, to the rest of the body, by tiny threads. Collagen's ability to hold water is what gives our skin its supple elasticity and youthful-looking appearance.

But all good things must come to an end – as the saying goes, and natural ageing begins on the day we are born and ends the day we die. As we age, so those collagen fibres lose their ability to hold water. They harden, degenerate and shift position and cause 'depressions' to form on the surface of the skin. What you've got now are wrinkles, furrows, lines and crows' feet. Some people find this degenerative process an intolerable occurrence – suddenly, that once young face has aged noticeably, and women in their thirties and forties in particular, not helped by media pressure to 'keep young and beautiful', tend to be the ones who worry about their fading looks the most.

COLLAGEN REPLACEMENT THERAPY: THE ANSWER FOR AGEING AND ACNE SCARRING?

You may have heard talk about collagen replacement therapy – and its ability to fill in the grooves of those wrinkles and restore the face to its former glory. But what exactly happens?

A mixture of highly purified bovine collagen, local anaesthetic and saline is injected into the skin using very fine needles. The saline is then absorbed, and the collagen eventually condenses into the areas where your own collagen has been depleted, thus cushioning up those depressions or wrinkles. But before therapy goes ahead, a test dose of collagen is injected into the skin in the forearm, at least a month before any other treatment takes place. In about 3% of cases there is an allergic reaction and treatment doesn't proceed. Collagen replacement therapy is given by trained practitioners, doctors, dentists and nurses.

How can it help wrinkles?
Collagen produces a temporary 'lifting' to lines along the upper lip, forehead grooves, those which run from your nose to your mouth, and frown lines between your eyebrows. It can also fill out crows' feet, though not so that they disappear entirely. It's a popular treatment – some 40,000 people have had collagen replacement therapy in this country alone.

How long does it last and what does it cost?
The effects of the therapy are rather short-lived. Six months to a year is the longest you can expect the treatment to last: around the mouth, the collagen disintegrates more quickly, because you use your mouth more frequently than, for

example, your forehead. This makes it an expensive anti-ageing treatment – with costs worked out per syringe/cc used. The average treatment for obvious lines would cost around £400, but if you were having most of your lines plumped up – even the tiny ones, it could cost around £900. Top-ups after a few months would cost a lot less and would last as long, providing there is still a bedrock of the existing collagen left in your skin. Eventually, the collagen breaks down and gets absorbed into the body – but it is not harmful. There is currently research into a longer lasting collagen solution which may appear on the market over the next twelve months. This type of collagen would last closer to a year.

Does it hurt?
An anaesthetic cream is applied to the area of your face to be injected, about half an hour before the needles are used. The nurse will make a series of tiny punctures into the skin, each delivering a tiny droplet of collagen. A small white weal will appear almost immediately, to show that the collagen has been correctly placed just below the surface of the skin. Round the mouth, where you are more sensitive anyway, the injections can be really quite painful, though the pain disappears pretty quickly. Your skin will feel puffy afterwards, and there may be some surface bruising which will disappear after seven days or so. Aloe vera gel can soothe any tender bits, and you should avoid make-up for a few hours. The end result is subtle but certainly effective. Friends won't know you've had treatment, though they will probably know that something is different about you. Maybe they'll think you've had a long luxurious holiday – or you're in love – something must have happened to give you that youthful glow!

How can collagen help people with skin problems?
Susie's story

Susie suffered from chronic **acne** during her teen years –
and this left her with noticeable scarring to her face. This
made her feel terribly self-conscious, as she so vividly
describes:

'You think when you're a teenager that your life will
turn around when the acne goes. But I never accounted for
the fact that I would be left with such noticeable scarring.
I felt ugly and an outcast. I got obsessed with looking at
everyone else's skin – comparing it to my own, hating
models with their fabulously smooth complexions. I
stopped socialising – I mistrusted any man who talked to
me, and never believed anyone could find me attractive. I
felt shy in the company of men, and all because I thought
my skin didn't measure up!

'It was someone at a beauty salon who recommended
collagen to me. I'd gone there for an aromatherapy massage,
and she told me that collagen replacement therapy could
help reduce the depth of my scars and smooth the skin. I felt
it was worth giving it a go, and was amazed at the results.
I've had a couple of top-ups over the year and it has
completely transformed me. I don't have to wear thick
make-up, I feel happy to meet people, my skin looks smooth
for the first time in years; it's the best thing I've ever done
for myself.'

Collagen is a simple and effective way to soften facial
scarring if, of course, you can afford it. Again, the skin will
return to its original condition over a period of time, and
top-ups will be necessary – but for dramatic results, it may
well be worth considering. Unfortunately though, for the
really deeper 'pitted' type of acne scar depression, collagen
won't work effectively.

For details of practitioners in your area, call the Collagen Information Service on 0800 888000.

OTHER WAYS TO REDUCE ACNE SCARRING

There are other ways to reduce acne scarring, which at the same time will help remove fine lines and the appearance of ageing. However, some of these are painful and dramatic processes, and you should think carefully before agreeing to undertake treatment, and only then, in the hands of a qualified expert. Recovery time is lengthy, so you need to take that into account as well – can you take that much time off work? Could you stand the pain?

Dermabrasion
This is quite a dramatic treatment, carried out under general anaesthetic, but it is effective for the deeper, more 'pitted' form of acne scarring. It involves removing the epidermis and the upper layer of the dermis using a high-powered rotation brush made of wire, or a diamond-covered sanding drum – it's a bit like sanding down a wall only of course, a thousand times more painful. After treatment, scabs form, and painkillers are needed. Ten days later, the scabs start to come away, revealing new skin underneath. It takes about ten days for the 'horror movie' look to go, and about a month for the swelling to subside, and the new skin will be extremely sun-sensitive. In many ways, it's a bit like a baby's skin. The advantages are high: removal of scarring and also wrinkles and fine lines, but the disadvantages are great too: an enormously long recovery period, a lot of pain, and a hugely sensitive skin.

Chemical face peeling

The aim of face peeling is to renew the supportive structure
of the skin and reduce age lines and wrinkles. It is also said
to be suitable for faces that have been left with severe skin
scarring. A chemical solution is applied to the skin while you
are sedated, and this penetrates down into the dermis,
where it acts to rearrange the collagen and elastin fibres,
and give the skin more elasticity and tightness. The solution
also removes dead cells from the surface of the skin by
literally burning the epidermis. As happens with any burning, the old skin peels back to reveal new pink tissue
underneath. This is a painful and, I feel, frightening treatment. Your skin will look peculiar during the recovery
phase, and will itch like mad. It is important not to scratch it,
as you could damage the new skin – and end up with scars
yet again. Your face will also take on a rosy hue for around
three months. Certainly the results are impressive, but at a
price.

Retin-A

Retin-A – a derivative of vitamin A – is used as a cure for
severe cases of acne. But there is more to this preparation
than meets the eye.

Retin-A was first invented by a leading American dermatologist called Professor Albert Kligman. Kligman
found that the derivative successfully cleared acne-prone
skin. At the same time, he discovered it could also smooth
out the skin, and even remove small surface wrinkles
around the eyes and on the cheeks. In trials, Retin-A also
seemed to have a marked improvement on deeper expression lines. As you can imagine, the cosmetics industry
viewed the findings with alarm. Here was a preparation,
available on prescription, which could potentially knock

out the whole anti-ageing beauty business. Since the late 1980s, a number of cosmetic companies have incorporated retinoids into their creams, but the problem with many over-the-counter remedies, like the latest fad for incorporating alpha-hydroxy acids and glycolic acids into creams, is that many simply do not contain enough to make a marked difference on the skin.

In some ways, this has to be welcomed, and you may recall a while back that Procter & Gamble pulled two products which contained these acids: New Skin Discovery from Oil of Ulay, and Response Cream from Max Factor, after customers complained the creams made their eyes tingle and water, and in some cases caused blurred vision. Retin-A, too, is an acid, and when you put it on the skin, it metabolises and gets down to work on the dermis where it supposedly harmlessly reduces the distortions caused by ageing.

I tried Retin-A myself about five years ago. I was researching an article into the beauty business, and purchased a bottle of the preparation in Harley Street for £100. I have delicate skin, which is prone to fine lines. I gave up using the preparation after just two weeks, because my skin became itchy, sore and flaky. I'm not saying that Retin-A doesn't work, though it didn't for my skin. I just feel it won't suit every skin type, and certainly not pale fine skins like mine.

Another important consideration is that most people who apply Retin-A find they can no longer tolerate natural sunlight – and I'm not talking about harsh sun. Even the slightest feeling of natural warmth on the skin will make it sting.

AHAs and glycolic acids
We all know that Cleopatra used to bathe in asses' milk – well, it seems she was on to a good thing as far as her skin

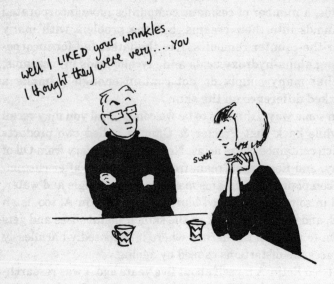

well I LIKED your wrinkles. I thought they were very.....you

sweet

was concerned. AHAs or fruit acids and glycolic acids are naturally occurring substances which you find in citrus fruits, milk and sugar cane. They work on the skin in the same way as a chemical facial peel – only much less dramatically. Used regularly, they have an effective exfoliating action – in other words, they strip the waxy substance that holds dead skin cells together on the surface of the skin, and in so doing, they produce a faster cell turnover. Getting rid of the dead cells is important, since old cells prevent the skin from taking up moisture, and the result is dry, rough, dehydrated-looking skin. In theory, these acids exfoliate the skin more effectively than any facial scrub, washing grains or loofah, with the result that the skin is fresh and rejuvenated. Glycolics differ from AHAs in that they speed up the process of dead skin removal and appear to be less aggressive to use.

Having said that, and in the light of Procter & Gamble's withdrawal of two products, these acids need to be treated with a certain degree of caution. Some dermatologists are questioning the continual paring down of the skin's surface through scrubs, acids and peels. The thought is that overuse could lead to a thinner skin, which is more prone to sensitivity and damage, ironically, from premature ageing. If in doubt, you should consult your GP before using these products.

CHAPTER 15

Your Home and Your Skin

The saying goes: 'You are what you eat' – well, in many ways, the same could be said for how and where you live. Unfortunately, suffering from a skin problem means that you are going to have to be extra careful about things like dust, detergents, bedding, sun, central heating, even clothing – in order to avoid exacerbating your condition. This is particularly relevant for **allergy-linked skin conditions**.

Rest assured, you won't have to turn into a fanatical Mrs Mop in order to achieve the right environment for your skin. That may have been true in the past, but now there are specialist companies who stock appropriate cleaners, bedding and filters, specifically geared to your needs. Prices are comparable to shop-bought standard products but the rest is down to changing your workaday habits: wearing rubber (or if you are sensitive to rubber, hypo-allergenic) gloves for washing up, as an example.

General life-style tips for dry and itchy skin conditions
• Keep the bedroom cool at night – a hot environment is more likely to make the skin itch.
• Wear household gloves to protect the hands. Cotton linings prevent sweating. Hypo-allergenic ones can replace rubber gloves, or wear cotton 'inners' in rubber gloves for

washing up. Keep gloves regularly clean and turn inside out to dry.

• In cold weather, always protect your hands with warm gloves.

• Protect exposed areas of skin with suitable emollients.

• If biological washing powders aggravate your skin condition, change to one specially formulated for sensitive skin. Perfumes in washing powders and fabric softeners can irritate **eczema** and are best avoided. Those made for sensitive skin come unperfumed. Always rinse your clothes thoroughly.

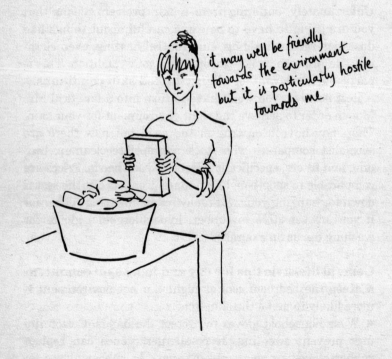

it may well be friendly towards the environment but it is particularly hostile towards me

- 'Green', environmentally friendly products don't necessarily mean kind to the skin.
- The chemicals used in swimming pools can be very drying – so shower well after a swim, and use an emollient cream or lotion afterwards.
- If your hands are dry, sensitive, itchy and sore, avoid peeling citrus fruits or chopping meat, onions, garlic or salty foods without using gloves. Likewise, don't wash your hair without gloves. You might find it useful to try the disposable gloves that are very fine and transparent and allow greater 'feel'; they are readily available from Boots and supermarkets. When you dry your hands, do so thoroughly, paying particular attention to in between the fingers.
- Use a humidifier or put a saucer of water on or next to radiators, to replenish lost moisture in the atmosphere.

AROUND THE HOUSE

House plants and the garden

Gardening can be problematic for those of you with **eczema** and sensitive skin – pesticides and even the soil itself can irritate. Wearing gloves again is essential, and to cut down on the amount of work you need to do in the garden, you might consider planting hardy perennials, or using forest bark to discourage weeds, as an example – or get your partner to do the digging!

Plants that can irritate the skin, especially **irritant contact dermatitis**, include: rue, primula obconica, geranium, cineraria and chrysanthemum. Choose your house plants with care and again avoid the above. House plants can trap dust and increase humidity – both of which can have a detrimental effect on **atopic eczema**.

161

Pets

As an avid cat lover, it breaks my heart to say this – but furry creatures aren't really to be recommended, especially if you have young children with **atopic eczema**, since cat and dog hairs can aggravate a number of skin conditions. Better to wait until your child has reached school age, and perhaps spend plenty of time with a dog or cat belonging to a friend, to see if any problems might occur before you buy your own. Fish are fine if you want a pet – they can even be quite soothing. Birds are out, since feathers can affect those of you with both asthma and **eczema**. For this reason too, you should avoid pillows and duvets filled with feathers; stick instead to a synthetic fibre.

Heating

Hot rooms fuelled by central heating can kick start a bad attack of the scratches. As soon as winter starts, and I'm back into socks and warm rooms, my legs itch and scale like mad! The answer is to turn the heating down a degree or two, get an ioniser and make sure that you put a saucer of

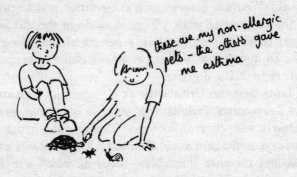

these are my non-allergic pets – the others gave me asthma

water near radiators. Avoided fan heaters, as they tend to blow dust particles about the house.

Water softeners
Hard water can really affect your skin, drying it out and irritating it still further. Water softeners are ideal as you will need to use less detergent for laundry and the water won't harm your skin so much. However, they are terribly expensive.

Dust mites
Children with **atopic eczema** in particular, benefit from living in as dust-free an environment as possible. This might sound a nightmarish scenario for a young mum to cope with, but there are steps you can take which will cut down on the chances of dust settling into impossible-to-get-at corners, and thus hopefully cut down on your workload. If you don't have fitted carpets, don't get them – a wooden floor or linoleum-covered floor is far better, since it is easier to keep really clean. The same goes for blinds as opposed to curtains. Curtains hide dust in their folds.

House dust mites and mould fungi are found in every household. Mites feed off skin scales, mould fungi and dust particles, although it is not the mite itself but its excrement which triggers allergic reactions. These minute particles get swept up into the air, inhaled into our lungs (particularly bad for asthmatic **eczema** sufferers), and land on our skin. The house dust mite has a lifespan of around four months, produces about 200 times its weight in excrement and lays up to 300 eggs – a real microscopic horror story! Dust mites thrive in warm, slightly dampish environments, and their favourite place of all is the bed. Here they find warmth and a plentiful supply of their number one food choice – human skin scales.

Keeping the bedroom free of dust mites

First off, the bed. Old mattresses tend to harbour millions of house dust mites, but the problem won't be solved by buying a new mattress, since they will soon colonise that as well. You can however get mattress covers and pillow covers specially designed for people who are allergic to dust mites. They cost about £35 for a double mattress, which is a lot cheaper than buying a new mattress! They allow moisture to escape, but are designed to trap the mites' faeces beneath their surface, thus reducing the number that can escape into the air.

You can also buy dust mite proofed pillows and duvets specially treated with Actigard, but obviously this can work out to be expensive. If you can't afford to start afresh with your laundry, make sure you regularly wash your sheets, blankets and pillows at temperatures above 58 degrees Centigrade – lower than this and the house mite can survive. With cotton sheets, you can easily boil-wash.

Air the bedroom daily. Throw the windows open (yes, even in winter!). Dust mites hate the cold. If you can, air the bedding out of the window too – it may look very Mediterranean to your neighbours, but you'll be saving your skin!

Vacuum regularly – if you can afford it, buy an anti-allergy vacuum cleaner. Recent controlled trials by a leading NHS chest hospital found that using an inefficient vacuum cleaner actually did more harm than good. The cleaner increased the airborne dust mite by about 400%. An efficient vacuum cleaner has a strong suction effect and an ability to retain even the minutest particles of dust.

As far as dusting generally is concerned, damp dusting is better than dry, since a damp cloth will pick up the dust more efficiently. If your child has a favourite fluffy toy, remember it too can harbour dust mites. Popping toys into the freezer overnight will be enough to destroy the mites.

Clothing

Wearing pure cotton next to the skin is best. It feels soothing, it allows the skin to breathe, and it is far less itchy than wool or synthetic fabrics. Some people with skin conditions find silk, polyester and soft acrylic fine to wear – basically, it is best to be guided by the feel of the material. If it doesn't feel harsh or scratchy, chances are you'll be able to live with it and in it. Look at the seams on the inside. Will they make your skin feel itchy? I have had to return numerous bras that have been so badly made, they exacerbated my dry skin condition. If you have trouble finding pure cotton clothing, contact the National Eczema Society for a list of stockists. Their address is at the back of the book.

As we mentioned in the first part of the book, jewellery can pose terrible trouble for those of you who are nickel allergic. If you are not sure about the nickel content of a piece of jewellery, you can buy a clear fluid which, when painted on the metal, will turn pink if nickel is present. Your GP can tell you where to find this solution.

Stockists

A number of specialist manufacturers stock anti-allergy bedding, vacuum cleaners, clothes, sprays, etc. and will send you a brochure free of charge. Try the Healthy House, Cold Harbour, Ruscombe, Stroud, GL6 6DA. Tel: 01453 752216.

Bibliography

Acne – Advice on Clearing your Skin, Professor Ronald Marks, Methuen Australia, 1984.

Beat Psoriasis the Natural Way, Sandra Gibbons, Thorsons, 1992.

Changing Faces – the Challenge of Facial Disfigurement, James Partridge, Changing Faces, 1994.

The Complete Book of Beauty Treatments, Sandra Sedgbeer, Thorsons, 1994.

The Complete Book of Relaxation Techniques, Jenny Sutcliffe, Headline, 1991.

Coping with Psoriasis, Professor Ronald Marks, Sheldon Press, 1981.

Diets to Help Psoriasis, Harry Clements, Thorsons, 1993.

Eczema and Dermatitis – How to Cope with Inflamed Skin, Professor Rona MacKie, Dunitz, 1983.

Evening Primrose Oil, Liz Earle, Boxtree, 1994.

Handbook of Over-the-Counter Medicines, Dr Mike Smith, Kyle Cathie, 1993.

HEA Guide to Complementary Medicine and Therapies, Anne Woodham, 1994.

The Healing Power of Herbs, Michael T. Murray, Prima, 1992.

Healthy Skin – the Facts, Rona M. MacKie, Oxford University Press, 1992.

Herbs for Health, Liz Earle, Boxtree, 1994.

Skin Conditions, Hasnain Walji & Dr Andrea Kingston, Headway Healthwise, 1994.

The Skin Game, Gerald McKnight, Sidgwick & Jackson, 1989.

Skin Troubles, Leon Chaitow, Thorsons, 1987.

Superskin, Kathryn Marsden, Thorsons, 1993.

Which? Medicine, Rosalind Grant, Which? Books, 1992.

Which? Way to a Healthier Diet, Judy Byrne, Which? Books, 1993.

Your Skin, Dr Graham Colver, Harrap, 1990.

Useful Addresses

Acne Support Group
PO Box 230
Hayes
Middx UB4 9HW

British Homeopathic Association
27a Devonshire Street
London W1N 1RJ

Changing Faces
27 Cowper Street
London EC2A 4AP

Chi Clinic
10 Greycoat Place
Victoria
London SW1P 1SB

Cosmetic Camouflage Service
28 Worple Road
London SW19 4EE

The Council for Acupuncture
179 Gloucester Place
London NW1 6DX

Imperial Cancer Research Fund
PO Box 123
Lincoln's Inn Fields
London WC2A 3PX

International Federation of Aromatherapists
Stamford House
2–4 Chiswick High Road
London W4 1TH

National Eczema Society
163 Eversholt Street
London NW1 1BU

National Institute of Medical Herbalists
56 Longbrook Street
Exeter EX4 6AH

The Psoriasis Association
7 Milton Street
Northampton NN2 7JG

The Register of Chinese Herbal Medicine
PO Box 400
Wembley
Middx HA9 9NE

The Register of Qualified Aromatherapists
PO Box 6941
London N8 9HF

The Royal London Homeopathic Hospital
Great Ormond Street
London WC1N 3HR

Skinship UK
10 Thurstable Way
Tollesbury
Nr Maldon
Essex CM9 8SQ

Vitiligo Society
19 Fitzroy Square
London W1P 5HQ

Index

Headline Health Kicks

THE PRIME OF YOUR LIFE
Self help during menopause   Pamela Armstrong   £5.99 ☐

STOP COUNTING SHEEP
Self help for insomnia sufferers   Dr Paul Clayton   £5.99 ☐

AM I A MONSTER, OR IS THIS PMS?
Self help for PMS sufferers   Louise Rhoddon   £4.99 ☐

GET UP AND GO!
Self help for fatigue sufferers   Anne Woodham   £5.99 ☐

You can kick that problem!

All Headline books are available at your local bookshop or newsagent, or can be ordered direct from the publisher. Just tick the titles you want and fill in the form below. Prices and availability subject to change without notice.

Headline Book Publishing, Cash Sales Department, Bookpoint, 39 Milton Park, Abingdon, OXON, OX14 4TD, UK. If you have a credit card you may order by telephone – 01235 400400.

Please enclose a cheque or postal order made payable to Bookpoint Ltd to the value of the cover price and allow the following for postage and packing:

UK & BFPO: £1.00 for the first book, 50p for the second book and 30p for each additional book ordered up to a maximum charge of £3.00.
OVERSEAS & EIRE: £2.00 for the first book, £1.00 for the second book and 50p for each additional book.

Name ....

Address ....

....

....

If you would prefer to pay by credit card, please complete:
Please debit my Visa/Access/Diner's Card/American Express (delete as applicable) card no:

Signature .... Expiry Date ....